AF577389

Cardiac Drug Eruptions and Interactions

Cardiac Drug Eruptions and Interactions

JEROME Z. LITT, MD

Assistant Clinical Professor of Dermatology
Case Western Reserve University School of Medicine
Cleveland, Ohio

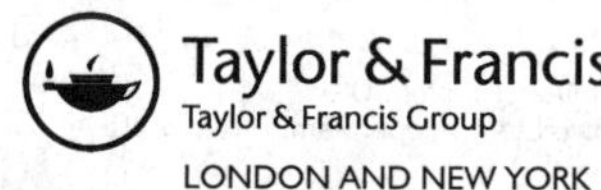

LONDON AND NEW YORK

©2005 Taylor & Francis, an imprint of the Taylor & Francis Group

First published in the United Kingdom in 2005
by Taylor & Francis,
an imprint of the Taylor & Francis Group,
2 Park Square, Milton Park
Abingdon, Oxon OX14 4RN, UK

Tel +44 (0) 20 7017 6000
Fax: +44 (0) 20 7017 6699
Website: www.tandf.co.uk

All rights reserved. No part of this publication may be reproduced, stored in a retrieval system, or transmitted, in any form or by any means, electronic, mechanical, photocopying, recording, or otherwise, without the prior permission of the publisher or in accordance with the provisions of the Copyright, Designs and Patents Act 1988 or under the terms of any licence permitting limited copying issued by the Copyright Licensing Agency, 90 Tottenham Court Road, London W1P 0LP.

Although every effort has been made to ensure that all owners of copyright material have been acknowledged in this publication, we would be glad to acknowledge in subsequent reprints or editions any omissions brought to our attention.

British Library Cataloguing in Publication Data

Data available on application

Library of Congress Cataloguing-in-Publication Data

Data available on application

ISBN 1-84184-602-3

Distributed in North and South America by
Taylor & Francis
2000 NW Corporate Blvd
Boca Raton, FL 33431, USA

Within Continental USA
Tel: 800 272 7737; Fax: 800 374 3401
Outside Continental USA
Tel: 561 994 0555; Fax: 561 361 6018
E-mail: orders@crcpress.com

Distributed in the rest of the world by
Thomson Publishing Services
Cheriton House
North Way
Andover, Hampshire SP10 5BE, UK
Tel: +44 (0) 1264 332424
E-mail: salesorder.tandf@thomsonpublishingservices.co.uk

Composition by AMA DataSet Limited, Preston, UK
Printed and bound by Antony Rowe Ltd., Chippenham, Wiltshire, UK

CONTENTS

INTRODUCTION

Any drug can cause any rash.

According to the World Health Organization, an adverse reaction (ADR) – or adverse event (ADE) – to a drug has been defined as any noxious or unintended reaction to a drug that has been administered in standard doses by the proper route for the purposes of prophylaxis, diagnosis, or treatment. This definition does not include abuse, overdose, withdrawal, or error of administration. While most eruptions are mild and self-limited, severe and life-threatening eruptions do occur, as seen in Torsades de pointes and Stroke. Death is the ultimate adverse drug event, and has now been incorporated into the book.

ADRs are underreported and thus are an underestimated cause of morbidity and mortality. The incidence and severity of ADRs can be influenced by age, sex, disease, genetic factors, type of drug, route of administration, duration of therapy, dosage, and bioavailability, as well as interactions with other drugs. It has been estimated that fatal ADRs are the third or fourth leading cause of death in the US.

This Pocketbook of Cardiologic Drug Eruptions and Interactions describes and catalogs the adverse effects of **over 160** commonly prescribed and over-the-counter generic drugs and herbals used in cardiology or having cardiovascular side effects. These drugs include classes such as ACE inhibitors, Alpha and Beta adrenoreceptor agonists, Antiarrhythmic agents, Anticoagulants, Antidiabetic agents, Antihypertensives, Antiplatelets, Calcium channel blockers, Carbonic anhydrase inhibitors, Diuretics, Hypolipidemic agents, Sulfonamide derivatives, Thrombolytics, and Vasodilators. The drugs have been listed and indexed by both their **Generic** and **Trade** (**Brand**) names for easy accessibility.

In addition to adverse drug reactions, there are many severe, hazardous **interactions** between two or more drugs. I have incorporated only the clinically important, potentially hazardous drug interactions that can trigger potential harm, and could be life-threatening. These interactions are predictable and well documented in controlled studies; they should be avoided.

For each drug, I have listed the known adverse side effects – in the form of drug reactions – that can develop from the use of the corresponding drug. These include those involving the skin, hair, nails, eyes, hematopoietic and mucous membrane side effects. The section entitled 'other' includes such reactions as tinnitus, serotonin syndrome, depression, rhabdomyolysis, insomnia, and death.

The first part of the book lists, in alphabetical order, the **Generic** and **Trade name** drugs with their corresponding names for easy access to the **A–Z** section – the main body of the book. Next comes a listing of the various **Classes** of drugs, and those **Generic** drugs that belong to each class. The last part of the book includes listings of common cardiology reactions caused mainly by non-cardiology drugs.

The major portion of the Pocketbook – the body of the work – lists the Generic drugs, herbals and supplements in alphabetical order and the adverse reactions that can arise from their use. The numbers in square brackets refer to the number of references recorded for each reaction. These references are available on my website (www.drugeruptiondata.com) or in the latest edition of the Drug Eruption Reference Manual.

USAGE, STYLE & CONVENTIONS EMPLOYED IN THIS POCKETBOOK

The **Generic Drug** name is at the top of each page.

The **Trade (Brand) Name(s)** are then listed alphabetically. When there are many **Trade Names**, the ten (or so) most commonly recognized ones are listed. This compilation lists and cross-references both the **Trade *and* Generic** names of all the cataloged drugs. Following the more common **Trade Name** drugs are recorded – in parentheses – the latest name of the pharmaceutical company that is marketing the drug.

Beneath the **Trade Name** listing is a list of Other **Common Trade Names**, those drugs from other countries. Then appear the **Indication(s)**, the **Category** in which the drug belongs, and the **Half-Life** of each drug, when known, and the **Potentially hazardous interactions** between drugs. On occasion, an important or pertinent **Note** will follow.

Reactions: These are the **Adverse Reactions** to the particular **Generic** drug. They are classified into **Categories: Skin, Hair, Nails, Hematopoietic, Eyes**, and **Other**. (**Other** refers to **Mucous Membrane, Teeth, Muscle** and various other **Reactions**.) **Reactions** are listed alphabetically under each heading. Alongside each **Reaction Pattern** are square bracketed numbers that refer to the number of references in the main Drug Eruption Reference Manual and my website. Numbers in round brackets refer to the incidence of the reaction, e.g. (3 cases) or (15%).

In the case of **herbals** and **supplements**, the format is slightly different. The herbals feature the scientific species and genus, purported indications and other uses. Then follows the same format as the generic drugs.

There are occasions when there are very few adverse reactions to a specific drug. These drugs are still included, since there is often **positive significance in negative findings**.

Jerome Z. Litt, M.D.
February, 2005

INDEX OF GENERIC AND TRADE NAMES

Generic drug names are in **bold**

CLASSES OF DRUGS

ACE inhibitors
benazepril
candesartan*
captopril
enalapril
eprosartan*
fosinopril
irbesartan*
lisinopril
losartan*
moexipril
olmesartan
perindopril
quinapril
ramipril
telmisartan*
trandolapril
valsartan*
*Angiotenin II receptor antagonist

Alpha adrenergic receptor inhibitors
brimonidine
dexmedetomidine
doxazosin
methyldopa
phenoxybenzamine
phentolamine
phenylephrine
prazosin
tamsulosin
terazosin
tolazoline

Alpha adrenoreceptor agonists
apraclonide
clonidine
guanabenz
guanethidine
guanfacine
mirtazapine
tizanidine

Antiarrhythmic agents and class
acebutolol
adenosine
amiodarone III
atropine
bretylium III
chlorothiazide
digoxin
diltiazem IV
disopyramide IV
dofetilide III
edrophonium
esmolol II
flecainide IC
ibutilide III
isoproterenol
lidocaine IB
metoprolol
mexiletine IB
minoxidil
moricizine IA
phenytoin IB
procainamide IA
propafenone IC
propranolol II
quinidine IA
sotalol III
tocainide IB
verapamil IV

Anticoagulants [1]
Antiplatelets [2]
Thrombolytics [3]
abciximab [2]
alteplase [3]
anagrelide [2]
anisindione [1]

anistreplase [3]
argatroban [1]
aspirin [2]
bivalirudin [1]
cilostazol [2]
clopidogrel [2]
dalteparin [1]
danaparoid [1]
dicumarol [1]
dipyridamole [2]
enoxaparin [1]
epitifibatide [2]
heparin [1]
protamine sulfate [1]
reteplase [3]
streptokinase [3]
tenecteplase [3]
ticlodipine [2]
tinzaparin [1]
torsemide [1]
urokinase [3]
warfarin [1]

Antidiabetic agents

acarbose
acetohexamide
chlorpropamide
glimepiride
glipizide
glucagon
glyburide
insulin
metformin
miglitol
nateglinide
pioglitazone
repaglinide
rosiglitazone
tolazamide
tolbutamide

Antihypertensives

acebutolol
amiloride
amlodipine
atenolol
benazepril
bendroflumethiazide
benzthiazide
betaxolol
bisoprolol
bumetanide
candesartan
captopril
carteolol
carvedilol
chlorothiazide
chlorthalidone
clonidine
cyclothiazide
diazoxide
diltiazem
doxazosin
enalapril
eplerenone
eprosartan
esmolol
ethacrynic acid
felodipine
fosinopril
furosemide
guanabenz
guanadrel
guanethidine
guanfacine
hydralazine
hydrochlorothiazide
hydroflumethiazide
indapamide
irbesartan
isradipine
labetalol
lisinopril
losartan
mecamylamine
meclofenamate
methyclothiazide
methyldopa

metolazone
metoprolol
minoxidil
moexipril
nadolol
nicardipine
nifedipine
nimodipine
nisoldipine
nitroglycerin
penbutolol
perindopril
phenoxybenzamine
phentolamine
pindolol
polythiazide
prazosin
propranolol
quinapril
quinethazone
ramipril
reserpine
spironolactone
telmisartan
terazosin
timolol
tolazoline
torsemide
trandolapril
triamterene
trichlormethiazide
valsartan
verapamil
yohimbine

Beta-blockers
acebutolol
atenolol
betaxolol
bisoprolol
carteolol
carvedilol
esmolol
labetalol
levobetaxolol
levobunolol
metipranolol
metoprolol
nadolol
penbutolol
pindolol
propranolol
sotalol
timolol

Calcium channel blockers
amlodipine
bepridil
diltiazem
enalapril
felodipine
isradipine
nicardipine
nifedipine
nimodipine
nisoldipine
trandolapril
verapamil

Diuretics
acetazolamude
amiloride
bendroflumethiazide
benzthiazide
bumetanide
chlorthalidone
chlorthiazide
cyclothiazide
ethacrynic acid
furosemide
hydrochlorothiazide
hydroflumethiazide
indapamide
isosorbide
methazolamide
methyclothiazide
metolazone

polythiazide
quinethazone
spironolactone
torsemide
triamterene
trichlormethiazide

Diuretics, loop
bumetanide
ethacrynic acid
furosemide
torsemide

Hypolipidemic agents HMG-CoA reductase inhibitors (statins)
atorvastatin
cholestyramine
clofibrate
colesevelam
colestipol
fenofibrate
fluvastatin
gemfibrozil
lovastatin
niacin
pravastatin
probucol
rosuvastatin
simvastatin

Sulfonamide derivatives
Diuretics carbonic anhydrase inhibitor
acetazolamide
methazolamide
Diuretics, loop
bumetanide
furosemide
torsemide
Diuretics, thiazide
bendroflumethiazide
benzthiazide
chlorothiazide
chlorthalidone
cyclothiazide
hydrochlorothiazide
hydroflumethiazide
indapamide
methyclothiazide
metolazone
polythiazide
quinethazone
trichlormethiazide
Hypoglycemic agents, oral
acetohexamide
chlorpropamide
glipizide
glyburide
tolazamide
tolbutamide

Vasodilators
hydralazine
isosorbide dinitrate
isoxsuprine
minoxidil
nesiritide
nitroglycerin
papaverine
tolazoline
treprostinil

ABCIXIMAB

Synonym: C7E3
Trade name: ReoPro (Lilly)
Indications: Thrombotic arterial disease
Category: Antiplatelet; Glycoprotein IIb/IIIa inhibitor
Half-life: 10–30 minutes – given intravenously
Clinically important, potentially hazardous interactions with: fondaparinux, reteplase

Reactions

Skin
- Acute generalized exanthematous pustulosis (AGEP)
- Cellulitis (0.3%)
- Edema [1]
- Peripheral edema (1.6%)
- Petechiae (0.3%)
- Pruritus (0.3%) [1]

Other
- Anaphylactoid reactions [3]
- Headache
- Hyperesthesia (1%)
- Injection-site reactions (3.6%)
- Myalgia (0.3%)

ACEBUTOLOL

Trade name: Sectral
Other common trade names: *Acecor; Acetanol; Alol; Apo-Acebutolol; Monitan; Neptal; Novo-Acebutolol; Nu-Acebutolol; Prent; Rhodiasectral; Rhotral*
Indications: Hypertension, angina, ventricular arrhythmias
Category: Antiarrhythmic; Antihypertensive; Beta-adrenoceptor blocker
Half-life: 3–7 hours
Clinically important, potentially hazardous interactions with: clonidine, verapamil

Note: Cutaneous side effects of beta-receptor blockaders are clinically polymorphous. They apparently appear after several months of continuous therapy. Atypical psoriasiform, lichen planus-like, and eczematous chronic rashes are mainly observed. (1983): Hödl St, *Z Hautkr* (German) 1:58, 17

Reactions

Skin
- Dermatitis
- Diaphoresis [1]
- Edema (1–10%)
- Erythema multiforme (<1%)
- Exanthems (4%) [1]
- Exfoliative dermatitis
- Facial edema (<1%)
- Hyperkeratosis (palms and soles)
- Lichenoid eruption [2]
- Lupus erythematosus (<1%) [12]
- Pigmentation
- Pityriasis rubra pilaris [1]
- Pruritus (<2%)
- Psoriasis [2]
- Rash (sic) (1–10%)
- Raynaud's phenomenon [2]
- Toxic epidermal necrolysis

Urticaria [1]
Vasculitis [2]
Xerosis

Hair

Hair – alopecia

Nails

Nails – dystrophy
Nails – onycholysis
Nails – pigmentation
Nails – pincer (reverse transverse curvature of the nails) [1]

Eyes

Oculo-mucocutaneous syndrome [1]

Other

Dysgeusia
Hyperesthesia (<2%)
Myalgia (1–10%)
Oral lichenoid eruption
Peyronie's disease [1]
Xerostomia (<1%)

ACETAZOLAMIDE

Trade name: Diamox (Wyeth)
Other common trade names: *Acetazolam; Ak-Zol; Dazamide; Defiltran; Diuramid; Novo-Zolamide*
Indications: Epilepsy, glaucoma
Category: Anticonvulsant; Carbonic anhydrase inhibitor; Sulfonamide diuretic
Half-life: 2–6 hours
Clinically important, potentially hazardous interactions with: ephedra, lithium

Reactions

Skin

Acute generalized exanthematous pustulosis (AGEP) [2]
Bullous eruption (<1%) [1]
Erythema multiforme [2]
Exanthems [2]
Frostbite [1]
Lupus erythematosus [1]
Photosensitivity
Pruritus
Purpura [1]
Pustular psoriasis [1]
Pustules [1]
Rash (sic) (<1%)
Rosacea [1]
Stevens–Johnson syndrome
Toxic epidermal necrolysis (<1%) [1]
Urticaria

Hair

Hair – hirsutism [1]

Hematopoietic

Thrombocytopenia [1]

Other

Ageusia
Anaphylactoid reactions [3]
Anosmia
Dysgeusia (>10%) (metallic taste) [3]
Extravasation [1]
Headache
Myalgia [1]
Paresthesias (<1%) [1]
Tinnitus
Xerostomia (<1%)

***Note:** Acetazolamide is a sulfonamide and can be absorbed systemically. Sulfonamides can produce severe, possibly fatal, reactions such as toxic epidermal necrolysis and Stevens–Johnson syndrome

ACETOHEXAMIDE

Trade name: Dymelor (Barr)
Other common trade names: *Dimelin; Dimelor*
Indications: non-insulin dependent diabetes type II
Category: Oral hypoglycemic; Sulfonylurea antidiabetic
Half-life: 1–6 hours

Reactions

Skin
- Diaphoresis
- Eczema
- Erythema (<1%)
- Exanthems (<1%)
- Lichenoid eruption
- Photosensitivity (1–10%)
- Pruritus (<1%)
- Rash (sic) (1–10%)
- Urticaria (1–10%)

Hair
- Hair – alopecia [1]

Other
- Headache
- Paresthesias
- Porphyria cutanea tarda

***Note:** Acetohexamide is a sulfonamide and can be absorbed systemically. Sulfonamides can produce severe, possibly fatal, reactions such as toxic epidermal necrolysis and Stevens–Johnson syndrome

ADENOSINE

Trade names: Adenocard (Fujisawa); Adenoscan (King)
Other common trade names: *Adenic; Adeno-Jec; Adenocur; Adenoject; Adrecar; Atp; Krenosin; Krenosine*
Indications: Paroxysmal supraventricular tachycardia, varicose vein complications with stasis dermatitis
Category: Antiarrhythmic
Half-life: seconds
Clinically important, potentially hazardous interactions with: carbamazepine, dipyridamole, theophylline

Reactions

Skin
- Burning (<1%)
- Diaphoresis (<1%)
- Flushing (18%)
- Rash (sic)

Other
- Dizziness (1%)
- Dysgeusia (<1%)
- Headache
- Numbness (1%)
- Paresthesias (1%)
- Tendinitis

ALBUTEROL

Synonym: salbutamol
Trade names: AccuNeb (DEY); Combivent (Boehringer Ingelheim); Duoneb (DEY); Proventil (Schering); Ventolin (GSK); Volmax (Muro)
Other common trade names: *Asmaven; Broncho-Spray; Cobutolin; Salbulin; Ventoline*
Indications: Bronchospasm associated with asthma
Category: Beta-2-adrenergic agonist; Bronchodilator (sympathomimetic)
Half-life: 3–6 hours
Clinically important, potentially hazardous interactions with: atomoxetine, epinephrine

Combivent is albuterol and ipratropium

Reactions

Skin
- Angioedema
- Chills
- Dermatitis [1]
- Diaphoresis (1–10%) [1]
- Erythema (palmar) (with infusion) [2]
- Exanthems
- Flushing (1–10%)
- Lupus erythematosus (pseudo-lupus) [1]
- Pallor
- Pruritus [1]
- Shaking
- Urticaria [1]

Other
- Dysgeusia (1–10%)
- Headache
- Tinnitus
- Tremor
- Xerostomia (1–10%)

ALFUZOSIN

Trade name: Uroxatral (Sanofi-Aventis)
Other common trade name: *Xatral*
Indications: Benign prostatic hyperplasia
Category: Alpha 1-adrenergic blocker
Half-life: 10 hours
Clinically important, potentially hazardous interactions with: atenolol, cimetidine, diltiazem, itraconazole, ketoconazole, ritonavir

Reactions

Skin
- Allergic reactions (sic) [1]
- Dermatomyositis [1]
- Rash (sic)
- Upper respiratory infection (3%)

Other
- Abdominal pain (1–2$)
- Chest pain
- Dizziness (6%) [6]
- Fatigue (3%)
- Headache (3%)
- Pain (1–2%)
- Pharyngitis (1–2%)
- Priapism
- Sinusitis (1–2%)

ALTEPLASE

Trade name: Activase (Genentech)
Other common trade names: *Actilyse; Activacin; Lysatec-rt-PA*
Indications: Acute myocardial infarction, acute pulmonary embolism
Category: Thrombolytic (tissue plasminogen activator)
Half-life: 30–45 minutes
Clinically important, potentially hazardous interactions with: nitroglycerin, ticlopidine

Reactions

Skin
Angioedema [4]
Purpura (<1%) [1]
Rash (sic) (<0.02%)
Urticaria (<1%) [1]

Hematopoietic
Ecchymoses (1–10%)

Other
Anaphylactoid reactions (<0.02%) [3]
Death [1]
Gingivitis (<1%)
Headache
Hypersensitivity [1]

AMILORIDE

Trade names: Midamor (Merck); Moduretic (Merck)
Other common trade names: *Amikal; Kaluril; Medamor; Midoride; Modamide; Nirulid; Ride*
Indications: Prevention of hypokalemia associated with kaliuretic diuretics, management of edema in hypertension
Category: Potassium-sparing antihypertensive diuretic
Half-life: 6–9 hours
Clinically important, potentially hazardous interactions with: benazepril, captopril, cyclosporine, enalapril, fosinopril, lisinopril, moexipril, quinapril, quinidine, ramipril, spironolactone, trandolapril

Moduretic is amiloride and hydrochlorothiazide

Reactions

Skin
Diaphoresis
Exanthems [1]
Flushing (>1%)
Photosensitivity [1]
Pruritus (<1%)
Purpura
Rash (sic) (<1%)
Urticaria
Vasculitis
Xerosis (<1%)

Hair
Hair – alopecia (<1%)

Other
Anaphylactoid reactions
Dysgeusia (<1%)
Gynecomastia (1–10%)
Headache
Paresthesias (<1%)

Tinnitus
Tremor
Xerostomia (<1%)

AMINOCAPROIC ACID

Trade name: Amicar (Xanodyne)
Other common trade names: *Capramol; Caproamin; Caprolisin; Ipron; Ipsilon; Resplamin*
Indications: To provide hemostasis in the treatment of fibrinolysis
Category: Antifibrinolytic; Hemostatic
Half-life: 1–2 hours

Reactions

Skin
Bullous eruption [1]
Dermatitis [3]
Eczema
Edema
Exanthems [1]
Kaposi's sarcoma
Pruritus
Purpura [2]
Purpura fulminans [1]
Rash (sic) (1–10%)
Urticaria

Other
Anaphylactoid reactions
Death [1]
Headache
Injection-site erythema
Injection-site phlebitis
Injection-site reactions (sic)
Muscle necrosis
Myalgia (1–10%) [1]
Rhabdomyolysis [9]
Thrombophlebitis
Tinnitus

AMIODARONE

Trade names: Cordarone (Wyeth); Pacerone (Upsher-Smith)
Other common trade names: *Aratac; Corbionax; Cordarex; Cordarone X; Tachydaron*
Indications: Ventricular fibrillation, ventricular tachycardia
Category: Class III antiarrhythmic
Half-life: 26–107 days
Clinically important, potentially hazardous interactions with: abarelix, amprenavir, anisindione, arsenic, ciprofloxacin, dicumarol, digoxin, diltiazem, enoxacin, fentanyl, fosamprenavir, gatifloxacin, **grapefruit Juice**, lomefloxacin, methotrexate, moxifloxacin, norfloxacin, ofloxacin, quinidine, rifabutin, rifampin, rifapentine, ritonavir, sparfloxacin, verapamil, warfarin

Reactions

Skin
Allergic reactions (sic) [1]
Angioedema [1]
Basal cell carcinoma [1]
Diaphoresis [2]
Edema (1–10%)

Erythema multiforme [1]
Erythema nodosum (<1%) [2]
Exanthems [5]
Exfoliative dermatitis [1]
Facial erythema (3.1%) [2]
Flushing (1–10%)
Iododerma [3]
Keratosis pilaris [1]
Linear IgA dermatosis [6]
Lupus erythematosus [4]
Photosensitivity (10–30%) [36]
Pigmentation [57]
Pruritus (1–5%) [2]
Psoriasis [2]
Purpura (2%) [1]
Pustular psoriasis [1]
Rash (sic) (<1%)
Rosacea [1]
Side effects (sic) [1]
Stevens–Johnson syndrome (<1%)
Toxic epidermal necrolysis [3]
Urticaria [1]
Vasculitis (<1%) [5]

Hair
Hair – alopecia (<1%) [6]
Hair – hypertrichosis [1]

Eyes
Dyschromatopsia [1]

Hematopoietic
Ecchymoses (<1%)

Other
Death [2]
Dysgeusia (1–10%) [1]
Headache
Paresthesias (4–9%)
Parosmia (1–10%)
Pseudoporphyria [1]
Pseudotumor cerebri (<1%)
Sialorrhea (1–3%)
Torsades de pointes [4]
Tremor

AMLODIPINE

Trade names: Lotrel (Novartis); Norvasc (Pfizer)
Other common trade names: *Amdepin; Amlodin; Amlogard; Amlopin; Amlor; Istin; Norvas*
Indications: Hypertension, angina
Category: Antianginal; Antihypertensive; Calcium channel blocker
Half-life: 30–50 hours
Clinically important, potentially hazardous interactions with: epirubicin, imatinib

Lotrel is amlodipine and benazepril

Reactions

Skin
Dermatitis (1–10%)
Diaphoresis (<1%)
Discoloration (<1%)
Edema (5–14%) [11]
Erythema multiforme [1]
Exanthems (2–4%) [1]
Flushing (1–10%) [4]
Granuloma annulare [1]
Lichen planus [1]
Lichenoid eruption [1]
Lupus erythematosus [1]
Peripheral edema (>10%) [8]
Petechiae (<1%)
Pruritus (2–4%) [4]
Purpura (<1%) [1]
Rash (sic) (1–10%)
Telangiectasia (facial) [3]

Urticaria (<1%)
Vasculitis [1]
Xerosis (<0.1%)

Hair

Hair – alopecia (<1%)

Hematopoietic

Thrombocytopenia [1]

Other

Acute intermittent porphyria [1]
Dysgeusia (<1%)
Gingival hypertrophy [13]
Gynecomastia [1]
Headache
Hyperesthesia (<1%)
Oral pigmentation [1]
Paresthesias (<1%)
Parkinsonism [2]
Parosmia (<0.1%)
Tendinitis [1]
Tinnitus
Tremor
Xerostomia (<1%)

AMYL NITRITE

Synonym: isoamyl nitrite
Trade name: Amyl Nitrite
Other common trade name: *Nitrit*
Indications: Angina pectoris
Category: Antianginal; Coronary vasodilator
Half-life: N/A
Clinically important, potentially hazardous interactions with: furosemide, sildenafil

Reactions

Skin

Allergic reactions (sic) [1]
Dermatitis [3]
Diaphoresis
Edema
Flushing (1–10%)
Pallor
Rash (sic) (<1%)

Other

Headache

ANAGRELIDE

Trade name: Agrylin (Shire)
Indications: Essential thrombocytopenia. To reduce elevated platelet count and the risk of thrombosis
Category: Phospholipase A 2 inhibitor; Platelet aggregation inhibitor
Half-life: ~3 days
Clinically important, potentially hazardous interactions with: fondaparinux

Reactions

Skin

Adverse effects (sic) (<5%)
Chills (<5%)
Edema (19.8%) [2]

Flu-like syndrome (<5%)
Peripheral edema (7.1%) [1]
Photosensitivity (<5%)
Pruritus (<5%)
Rash (sic) (7.8%)
Urticaria (7.8%)

Hair
Hair – alopecia (<5%)

Eyes
Visual hallucinations [1]

Hematopoietic
Ecchymoses (<5%)

Other
Aphthous stomatitis (<5%)
Arthralgia (<5%)
Back pain (6.4%)
Depression (<5%)
Headache
Leg cramps (<5%)
Myalgia (<5%)
Paresthesias (7.3%)
Tinnitus (<5%)

ANISINDIONE

Trade name: Miradon (Schering)
Indications: Adjunct in treatment of coronary occlusion, Atrial fibrillation
Category: Indanedione oral anticoagulant
Half-life: 3–5 days
Clinically important, potentially hazardous interactions with: amiodarone, bivalirudin, cimetidine, clofibrate, clopidogrel, cyclosporine, delavirdine, disulfiram, fluconazole, imatinib, itraconazole, ketoconazole, metronidazole, miconazole, penicillins, piperacillin, quinidine, quinine, rifabutin, rifampin, rifapentine, rofecoxib, sulfinpyrazone, testosterone, zileuton

Reactions

Skin
Chills
Dermatitis
Erythema
Erythema multiforme
Exanthems
Exfoliative dermatitis
Necrosis
Petechiae
Purple toe syndrome
Urticaria

Hair
Hair – alopecia

Hematopoietic
Ecchymoses

Other
Death
Hypersensitivity
Oral ulceration
Priapism
Stomatitis
Stomatodynia

ANISTREPLASE

Synonym: APSAC
Trade name: Eminase
Other common trade name: *Iminase*
Indications: Acute myocardial infarction
Category: Thrombolytic enzyme
Half-life: 70–120 minutes

Reactions

Skin
- Allergic reactions (sic)
- Angioedema
- Chills (<1%)
- Diaphoresis (<1%)
- Exanthems [1]
- Flushing
- Livedo reticularis [1]
- Purpura
- Rash (sic)
- Ulcerations [1]
- Urticaria [1]
- Vasculitis [5]

Hematopoietic
- Ecchymoses

Other
- Anaphylactoid reactions (1–10%) [1]
- Gingival hemorrhage
- Hypersensitivity [1]
- Myalgia [1]
- Serum sickness [1]

APRACLONIDINE

Trade name: Iopidine (Alcon)
Indications: Post-surgical intraocular pressure elevation
Category: Alpha-2-adrenoceptor stimulant; Sympathomimetic ophthalmic solution; Vasoconstrictor
Half-life: 8 hours

Reactions

Skin
- Allergic reactions (sic) (<1%) [5]
- Burning [1]
- Dermatitis (<1%) [3]
- Facial edema (<1%)
- Pruritus (10%) [1]
- Xerosis

Eyes
- Eyelid edema (<3%)
- Ocular inflammation [1]
- Periocular dermatitis [1]

Other
- Dysgeusia (3%)
- Headache
- Myalgia (0.2%)
- Paresthesias (<1%)
- Parosmia (0.2%)
- Xerostomia (1–10%) [1]

ARBUTAMINE

Trade name: GenESA (Sicor)
Indications: Diagnostic aid for coronary artery disease
Category: Adrenergic agonist; Nonradioactive diagnostic synthetic catecholamine
Half-life: 1.8 hours
Clinically important, potentially hazardous interactions with: abacavir, clidinium, clomipramine, desipramine, dicyclomine, digoxin, doxepin, flavoxate, glycopyrrolate, hyoscyamine, imipramine, mepenzolate, methantheline, nortriptyline, oxybutynin, procyclidine, propantheline, protriptyline, scopolamine, trihexyphenidyl, trimipramine

Reactions

Skin

Diaphoresis (1.5%)
Flushing (3%) [1]
Hot flashes (3%)
Rash (sic)

Other

Application-site reactions (0.1%)
Back pain (0.1%)
Cough (0.2%)
Dysgeusia (1.3%) [1]
Hyperesthesia (1.0%)
Pain (1.8%)
Paresthesias (2%)
Tremor (15%) [1]
Twitching (0.3%)
Xerostomia (1.1%)

ARGATROBAN

Trade name: Acova (GSK)
Indications: Heparin-induced thrombocytopenia
Category: Anticoagulant; Thrombin inhibitor
Half-life: 40–50 minutes
Clinically important, potentially hazardous interactions with: abacavir, butabarbital

Reactions

Skin

Allergic reactions (sic)
Bullous eruption (<1%)
Infections (4%)
Rash (sic) (<1%)

Other

Headache
Injection-site bleeding (2–5%)

ASPIRIN

Synonyms: acetylsalicylic acid; ASA
Trade names: Aggrenox (Boehringer Ingelheim); Alka-Seltzer; Anacin (Wyeth); Ascriptin (Novartis) (Wallace); Aspergum; Coricidin D; Darvon Compound (aaiPharma); Ecotrin (GSK); Empirin; Equagesic (Women First); Excedrin (Bristol-Myers Squibb); Fiorinal (Watson); Gelprin; Halfprin; Measurin; Norgesic (3M); Robaxisal; Soma Compound (MedPointe); Talwin Compound (Sanofi-Aventis); Vanquish
Other common trade names: *ASA; Aspro; ASS; Bex; Caprin; Claragine; Disprin; Ecotrin; Novasen; Rhonal*
Indications: Pain, fever, inflammation
Category: Nonsteroidal anti-inflammatory (NSAID) analgesic; Salicylate
Half-life: 15–20 minutes
Clinically important, potentially hazardous interactions with: bismuth, **boswellia**, **capsicum**, cholestyramine, **devil's claw**, dicumarol, etodolac, **evening Primrose**, **ginkgo biloba**, **ginseng**, heparin, ibuprofen, indomethacin, ketoprofen, ketorolac, methotrexate, **phellodendron**, **resveratrol**, reteplase, sermorelin, **sulfites**, tirofiban, urokinase, valdecoxib, valproic acid, verapamil, warfarin

Aggrenox is aspirin and dipyridamole

Reactions

Skin
- Acute generalized exanthematous pustulosis (AGEP) [1]
- Allergic reactions (sic) (<1%) (with dipyridamole) [1]
- Angioedema (1–5%) [21]
- Baboon syndrome [1]
- Bullous eruption (<1%) [4]
- Dermatitis herpetiformis [1]
- Dermatomyositis [1]
- Diaphoresis
- Erythema multiforme (<1%) [9]
- Erythema nodosum (<1%) [9]
- Erythroderma [1]
- Exanthems [11]
- Exfoliative dermatitis [1]
- Fixed eruption (<1%) [21]
- Flushing [1]
- Genital herpes [1]
- Graft-versus-host reaction [1]
- Granulomas [1]
- Herpes simplex [1]
- Lichenoid eruption [2]
- Parapsoriasis [1]
- Pemphigus [1]
- Petechiae [1]
- Photo-recall [1]
- Pigmented purpuric eruption [1]
- Pityriasis rosea [2]
- Pruritus [6]
- Psoriasis [2]
- Purpura [7]
- Pustular psoriasis [2]
- Rash (sic) (1–10%)
- Stevens–Johnson syndrome [4]
- Toxic epidermal necrolysis (<1%) [9]
- Ulcerations (<1%) (with dipyridamole)
- Urticaria (1–10%) [62]
- Vasculitis [3]

Hair
- Hair – alopecia [1]

Eyes
- Ocular hemorrhage [1]
- Periorbital edema [3]

Other

Ageusia (<1%) (with dipyridamole)
Anaphylactoid reactions (1–10%) [6]
Aphthous stomatitis [3]
Dysgeusia
Gingivitis (<1%) (with dipyridamole)
Headache
Hypersensitivity [3]
Myalgia (1.2%) (with dipyridamole)
Oral burn [1]
Oral lichen planus [1]
Oral mucosal eruption [3]
Oral ulceration [4]
Paresthesias (<1%) (with dipyridamole)
Pseudolymphoma [1]
Pseudoporphyria [1]
Tinnitus

ATENOLOL

Trade names: Tenoretic (AstraZeneca); Tenormin (AstraZeneca)
Other common trade names: *Antipressan; Apo-Atenol; AteHexal; Atendol; Evitocor; Noten; Novo-Atenol; Nu-Atenol; Taro-Atenol; Tenolin; Tenormine*
Indications: Angina, hypertension, acute myocardial infarction
Category: Antianginal; Antihypertensive; Beta-adrenoceptor blocker
Half-life: 6–7 hours (adults)
Clinically important, potentially hazardous interactions with: alfuzosin, clonidine, epinephrine, verapamil

Tenoretic is atenolol and chlorthalidone

Reactions

Skin

Acrocyanosis [1]
Dermatitis [1]
Diaphoresis
Edema
Erythema multiforme
Exanthems
Facial edema
Fixed eruption [1]
Grinspan's syndrome* [1]
Hyperkeratosis (palms and soles)
Lichenoid eruption [1]
Lupus erythematosus [2]
Necrosis [3]
Papulo-nodular lesions [1]
Photosensitivity
Pityriasis rubra pilaris [1]
Pruritus (1–5%)
Psoriasis [7]
Purpura
Pustular psoriasis [1]
Rash (sic) [1]
Raynaud's phenomenon [1]
Toxic epidermal necrolysis
Urticaria [2]
Vasculitis [1]
Vitiligo
Xerosis

Hair

Hair – alopecia [1]

Nails

Nails – dystrophy
Nails – onycholysis
Nails – pigmentation
Nails – splinter hemorrhages [1]

Eyes

Oculo-mucocutaneous syndrome [1]

Other
Anaphylactoid reactions [1]
Death [1]
Oral lichenoid eruption [1]
Peyronie's disease
Pseudolymphoma [1]

***Note:** Grinspan's syndrome: the triad of oral lichen planus, diabetes mellitus, and hypertension

ATORVASTATIN

Trade name: Lipitor (Pfizer)
Indications: Hypercholesterolemia
Category: Antihyperlipidemic; HMG-CoA reductase inhibitor
Half-life: 14 hours
Clinically important, potentially hazardous interactions with: azithromycin, bosentan, clarithromycin, cyclosporine, erythromycin, fosamprenavir, gemfibrozil, imatinib, itraconazole, niacin, telithromycin, verapamil

Reactions

Skin
Acne (<2%)
Allergic reactions (sic) (<2%)
Cheilitis (<2%)
Dermatitis (<2%)
Dermatomyositis [1]
Dermographism [1]
Diaphoresis (<2%)
Eczema (<2%)
Edema (<2%)
Exanthems
Facial edema (<2%)
Flu-like syndrome
Lichenoid eruption [1]
Linear IgA dermatosis [2]
Lymphocytic infiltration [1]
Petechiae (<2%)
Photosensitivity (<2%)
Pruritus (<2%) [1]
Rash (sic) (>3%) [1]
Seborrhea (<2%)
Toxic epidermal necrolysis [1]
Ulcerations (<2%)
Urticaria (<2%) [1]
Xerosis (<2%)

Hair
Hair – alopecia (<2%) [6]

Hematopoietic
Ecchymoses (<2%)

Other
Ageusia (<2%)
Death [1]
Dysgeusia (<2%)
Glossitis (<2%)
Gynecomastia (<2%)
Headache
Limb pain [1]
Myalgia (>3%) [13]
Myositis [2]
Oral ulceration (<2%)
Paresthesias (<2%)
Parosmia (<2%)
Polyneuropathy [2]
Rhabdomyolysis [9]
Stomatitis (<2%)
Tendinitis [1]

ATROPINE SULFATE

Trade names: Belladenal; Bellergal-S; Butibel; Donnagel; Donnatal; Donnazyme; Isopto Atropine; Lofene; Logen; Lomanate; Lomotil (Pfizer); Urised
Other common trade names: *Atropine Martinet; Atropt; Chibro-Atropine; Isopto; Tropyn Z; Vitatropine*
Indications: Salivation, sinus bradycardia, uveitis, peptic ulcer
Category: Anticholinesterase
Half-life: 2–3 hours

Reactions

Skin
Adverse effects (sic) [1]
Allergic reactions (sic) [2]
Bullous eruption [1]
Dermatitis [3]
Eccrine hidrocystomas [1]
Erythema (sheet-like)
Erythema multiforme (<1%) [2]
Exanthems
Exfoliative dermatitis [1]
Fixed eruption [2]
Flushing [1]
Hypohidrosis (>10%) [1]
Photosensitivity (1–10%)
Pruritus
Rash (sic) (<1%)
Stevens–Johnson syndrome [1]
Urticaria [1]
Xerosis

Eyes
Eyelid edema
Ocular allergic reactions (sic) [1]
Periocular dermatitis [3]

Other
Anaphylactoid reactions [1]
Dry mucous membranes [1]
Dysgeusia
Headache
Injection-site irritation (>10%)
Tremor
Xerostomia (>10%)

***Note:** Many of the above trade name drugs contain phenobarbital, scopolamine, hyoscyamine, hydrocodone, methenamine, etc

BENAZEPRIL

Trade names: Lotensin (Novartis); Lotensin-HCT (Novartis); Lotrel (Novartis)
Other common trade names: *Cibace; Cibacen; Cibacene*
Indications: Hypertension
Category: Angiotensin-converting enzyme (ACE) inhibitor; Antihypertensive
Half-life: 11–12 hours
Clinically important, potentially hazardous interactions with: amiloride, spironolactone, triamterene
Lotrel is benazepril and amlodipine; Lotensin-HCT is benazepril and hydrochlorothiazide

Reactions

Skin
- Angioedema (<1%) [6]
- Dermatitis
- Diaphoresis (<1%) [1]
- Exanthems [1]
- Flushing [1]
- Linear IgA dermatosis [1]
- Lupus erythematosus [1]
- Pemphigus foliaceus [1]
- Peripheral edema [1]
- Photosensitivity (<1%)
- Pruritus [1]
- Rash (sic) (<1%) [1]
- Urticaria [1]

Other
- Ageusia
- Cough [2]
- Dysgeusia [1]
- Headache
- Hypersensitivity
- Myalgia (<1%)
- Paresthesias (<1%)
- Tinnitus

BENDROFLUMETHIAZIDE

Trade names: Corzide (Monarch); Naturetin (Bristol-Myers Squibb)
Other common trade names: *Aprinox; Berkozide; Centyl; Naturine; Neo-Naclex; Pluryle*
Indications: Edema, diabetes insipidus, hypertension
Category: Antihypertensive; Thiazide diuretic
Half-life: 8.5 hours
Clinically important, potentially hazardous interactions with: digoxin, lithium

Corzide is bendroflumethiazide and nadolol

Reactions

Skin
- Allergic reactions (sic)
- Dermatitis [1]
- Diaphoresis
- Exanthems [1]
- Exfoliative dermatitis
- Facial edema
- Grinspan's syndrome** [1]
- Pemphigus
- Photosensitivity [1]
- Phototoxicity [2]
- Pruritus [1]
- Purpura
- Rash (sic)
- Urticaria
- Vasculitis

Hair
- Hair – alopecia

Eyes
- Dyschromatopsia

Other
- Anaphylactoid reactions
- Gynecomastia
- Paresthesias
- Tinnitus
- Xerostomia

***Note:** Bendroflumethiazide is a sulfonamide and can be absorbed systemically. Sulfonamides can produce severe, possibly fatal, reactions such as toxic epidermal necrolysis and Stevens–Johnson syndrome

****Note:** Grinspan's syndrome: the triad of oral lichen planus, diabetes mellitus, and hypertension

BENZTHIAZIDE

Trade names: Aquatag; Exna; Hydrex; Marazide; Proaqua
Other common trade names: *Diurin; Fovane; Regulon*
Indications: Hypertension
Category: Antihypertensive; Thiazide diuretic
Half-life: N/A
Clinically important, potentially hazardous interactions with: digoxin, lithium

Reactions

Skin
- Allergic reactions (sic) (<1%)
- Photosensitivity
- Purpura
- Rash (sic)
- Urticaria
- Vasculitis

Eyes
- Dyschromatopsia

Other
- Dysgeusia
- Paresthesias (<1%)

***Note:** Benzthiazide is a sulfonamide and can be absorbed systemically. Sulfonamides can produce severe, possibly fatal, reactions such as toxic epidermal necrolysis and Stevens–Johnson syndrome

BEPRIDIL

Trade name: Vascor (Ortho-McNeil)
Other common trade names: *Bapadin; Bepricol; Cordium; Cruor*
Indications: Angina pectoris
Category: Antianginal; Calcium channel blocker
Half-life: 24 hours
Clinically important, potentially hazardous interactions with: amprenavir, atazanavir, ciprofloxacin, enoxacin, epirubicin, fosamprenavir, gatifloxacin, lomefloxacin, **mistletoe**, moxifloxacin, norfloxacin, ofloxacin, ritonavir, sparfloxacin

Reactions

Skin
- Diaphoresis (<2%)
- Edema (1–10%)
- Irritation (sic)
- Peripheral edema (<1%)
- Rash (sic) (<2%) [1]

Other
- Dysgeusia (<1%)
- Myalgia (<1%)
- Paresthesias (2.5%)
- Tinnitus
- Torsades de pointes [1]
- Tremor (<9%)
- Xerostomia (1–10%) [2]

BETAXOLOL

Trade names: Betoptic [Ophthalmic] (Alcon); Kerlone (Pfizer)
Other common trade names: *Betoptic S; Betoptima; Kerlon; Optipres*
Indications: Open-angle glaucoma, hypertension
Category: Antihypertensive; Beta-adrenoceptor blocker
Half-life: 14–22 hours
Clinically important, potentially hazardous interactions with: clonidine, verapamil

Note: Cutaneous side effects of beta-receptor blockaders are clinically polymorphous. They apparently appear after several months of continuous therapy. Atypical psoriasiform, lichen planus-like, and eczematous chronic rashes are mainly observed. (1983): Hödl St, *Z Hautkr* 1:58, 17

Reactions

Skin
- Acne
- Allergic reactions (sic) (<2%)
- Angioedema
- Cold extremities
- Dermatitis [2]
- Diaphoresis (<2%)
- Edema (1.3%)
- Erythema (1–10%)
- Exanthems
- Exfoliative dermatitis
- Facial edema
- Flushing (<2%)
- Lupus erythematosus [1]
- Photosensitivity
- Pigmentation (palms) [1]
- Pruritus (1–10%)
- Psoriasis
- Purpura
- Rash (sic) (1.2%) [1]
- Raynaud's phenomenon
- Toxic epidermal necrolysis
- Urticaria
- Xerosis

Hair
- Hair – alopecia (following topical use) (<2%) [1]
- Hair – hypertrichosis (<2%)

Nails
- Nails – pigmentation (bluish)

Other
- Ageusia (<2%)
- Anaphylactoid reactions
- Depression [1]
- Dysgeusia (<2%)
- Glossitis (following topical use)
- Headache
- Mastodynia (<2%)
- Myalgia (3.2%)
- Myasthenia gravis [1]
- Oral ulceration (<2%)
- Paresthesias (1.9%)
- Peyronie's disease (<2%)
- Sialorrhea (<2%)
- Tinnitus
- Xerostomia (<2%)

BEVACIZUMAB

Trade name: Avastin (Genentech)
Indications: Colon cancer
Category: Angiogenesis inhibitor; Monoclonal antibody
Half-life: N/A

Reactions

Skin
Exfoliative dermatitis
Pigmentation
Ulcerations
Upper respiratory infection
Xerosis

Hair
Hair – alopecia

Nails
Nails – changes

Eyes
Lacrimation

Other
Abdominal pain
Asthenia
Dizziness
Dysgeusia
Headache
Myalgia
Oral ulceration
Pain
Stomatitis
Xerostomia

BISOPROLOL

Trade names: Zebeta (Barr); Ziac (Barr)
Other common trade names: *Concor; Cordalin; Detensiel; Emcor; Fondril; Monocor; Soprol*
Indications: Hypertension
Category: Beta-adrenoceptor blocker
Half-life: 9–12 hours

Ziac is bisoprolol and hydrochlorothiazide

Reactions

Skin
Acne
Angioedema
Diaphoresis (1%)
Eczema
Edema (3%)
Exanthems
Exfoliative dermatitis
Facial edema
Flushing
Lupus erythematosus
Peripheral edema (1–10%)
Photosensitivity
Pigmentation
Pruritus
Psoriasis
Purpura
Rash (sic) (1–10%)

Raynaud's phenomenon (1–10%)
Urticaria
Xerosis

Hair
Hair – alopecia

Nails
Nails – pigmentation

Other
Anaphylactoid reactions
Dysgeusia
Headache
Hyperesthesia (1.5%)
Myalgia (1–10%)
Paresthesias
Peyronie's disease
Tinnitus
Xerostomia (1.3%)

BIVALIRUDIN

Synonym: Hirulog
Trade name: Angiomax (The Medicines Company)
Indications: Angioplasty adjunct
Category: Anticoagulant; Thrombin inhibitor
Half-life: 25 minutes
Clinically important, potentially hazardous interactions with: anisindione, dicumarol, heparin, reteplase, streptokinase, tenecteplase, urokinase, warfarin

Reactions

Skin
Infections

Other
Back pain (42%)
Headache
Injection-site pain (8%)
Pain (15%)

BRETYLIUM

Other common trade names: *Bretylate; Critifib*
Indications: Ventricular tachycardia and fibrillation
Category: Antiarrhythmic class III
Half-life: 4–17 hours
Clinically important, potentially hazardous interactions with: arsenic, ciprofloxacin, enoxacin, gatifloxacin, lomefloxacin, moxifloxacin, norfloxacin, ofloxacin, sparfloxacin

Reactions

Skin
Diaphoresis (<1%)
Flushing (<1%)
Rash (sic) (<1%)
Side effects (sic) [1]

Other
Injection-site atrophy (<1%)
Injection-site necrosis (<1%)

BRIMONIDINE

Trade name: Alphagan (Allergan)
Indications: Open-angle glaucoma, ocular hypertension
Category: Alpha-2-adrenoceptor stimulant
Half-life: 12 hours

Reactions

Skin
- Allergic reactions (sic) (<1%) [2]
- Dermatitis [1]
- Upper respiratory infection (1–10%)

Nails
- Nails – lichen planus [1]

Eyes
- Blepharitis (1–10%)
- Eyelid crusting (1–10%)
- Eyelid edema (1–10%)
- Eyelid erythema (1–10%)
- Ocular allergy (sic) (4.2%) [4]
- Ocular burning (<10%) [4]
- Ocular erythema [1]
- Ocular pruritus (<10%)
- Ocular stinging (<10%) [4]
- Periocular dermatitis [1]
- Teardrop sign* [1]
- Uveitis [2]

Other
- Depression
- Dysgeusia (1–10%)
- Headache
- Hypersensitivity [2]
- Xerostomia (<10%) [6]

***Note:** The Teardrop sign is a laceration or deformity of the limbus of the eye

BUMETANIDE

Trade name: Bumex (Roche)
Other common trade names: *Bumedyl; Burinex; Fondiuran; Fontego; Lunetoron; Miccil; Primex*
Indications: Edema associated with congestive heart failure
Category: Antihypertensive; Sulfonamide loop diuretic
Half-life: 1–1.5 hours
Clinically important, potentially hazardous interactions with: amikacin, digoxin, gentamicin, kanamycin, neomycin, streptomycin, tobramycin

Reactions

Skin
- Allergic reactions (sic)
- Bullous eruption [1]
- Bullous pemphigoid [1]
- Dermatitis [1]
- Diaphoresis (0.1%)
- Erythema multiforme (<1%) [1]
- Exanthems
- Exfoliative dermatitis [1]
- Photosensitivity [1]
- Pruritus (<1%) [2]
- Purpura
- Rash (sic) (0.2%)
- Side effects (sic) (1.1%) [1]
- Urticaria (0.2%) [1]
- Vasculitis

Eyes

Periorbital edema (periorbital) [1]

Other

Headache

Nipple tenderness (0.1%)

Pseudoporphyria [1]

Xerostomia (0.1%)

***Note:** Bumetanide is a sulfonamide and can be absorbed systemically. Sulfonamides can produce severe, possibly fatal, reactions such as toxic epidermal necrolysis and Stevens–Johnson syndrome

CANDESARTAN

Trade name: Atacand (AstraZeneca)
Other common trade name: *Amias*
Indications: Hypertension
Category: Angiotensin II receptor antagonist; Antihypertensive
Half-life: 9 hours

Reactions

Skin

Angioedema [2]

Diaphoresis (>0.5%)

Edema

Exanthems (<1%)

Linear IgA dermatosis [1]

Peripheral edema (>1%)

Rash (sic) (>0.5%) [1]

Other

Cough [1]

Headache

Myalgia (>0.5%)

Paresthesias (>0.5%)

CAPTOPRIL

Synonym: ACE
Trade names: Capoten (Par); Capozide (Par)
Other common trade names: *Acenorm; Acepril; Adocor; APO-Capto; Captolane; Captoril; Lopirin; Lopril; Nu-Capto; Precaptil*
Indications: Hypertension
Category: Angiotensin-converting enzyme (ACE) inhibitor; Antihypertensive
Half-life: <3 hours
Clinically important, potentially hazardous interactions with: amiloride, spironolactone, triamterene

Capozide is captopril and hydrochlorothiazide

Reactions

Skin

Allergic reactions (sic) [2]

Angioedema (1–15%) [40]

Bullous eruption [1]

Bullous pemphigoid [3]

Dermatitis [3]

Erythroderma [2]
Exanthems (4–7%) [19]
Exfoliative dermatitis (<2%) [4]
Flushing (<1%) [2]
Graft-versus-host reaction [1]
Kaposi's sarcoma [2]
Lichen planus (pemphigoides) [1]
Lichenoid eruption [13]
Linear IgA dermatosis [5]
Lupus [1]
Lupus erythematosus [6]
Mycosis fungoides [2]
Palmar–plantar pustulosis [1]
Pemphigus (<2%) [21]
Pemphigus foliaceus [1]
Penile ulcers [2]
Photosensitivity [3]
Phototoxicity (<2%)
Pigmentation [2]
Pityriasis rosea (<2%) [6]
Pruritus (1–7%) [9]
Psoriasis [8]
Purpura [1]
Rash (sic) (4–7%) [11]
Stevens–Johnson syndrome [1]
Toxic epidermal necrolysis [3]
Urticaria [9]
Vasculitis [7]
Xerosis [1]

Hair
Hair – alopecia (<2%) [5]

Nails
Nails – dystrophy [2]
Nails – onycholysis [2]

Other
Ageusia (2–4%) [11]
Anaphylactoid reactions (during hemodialysis) [1]
Aphthous stomatitis (<2%) [4]
Cough [3]
Death
Dysgeusia (2–4%) (metallic or salty taste) [10]
Glossitis [3]
Glossopyrosis [1]
Gynecomastia [3]
Headache
Lymphadenopathy [1]
Myalgia
Oral burn [1]
Oral mucosal eruption [3]
Oral ulceration [3]
Paresthesias (<2%)
Pseudolymphoma [2]
Tongue ulceration [3]
Xerostomia (<2%)

CARTEOLOL

Trade name: Ocupress (ophthalmic) (Novartis)
Other common trade names: *Arteolol; Arteoptic; Calte; Carteol; Endak; Mikelan; Teoptic*
Indications: Glaucoma, hypertension
Category: Beta-adrenoceptor blocker
Half-life: 6 hours
Clinically important, potentially hazardous interactions with: clonidine, epinephrine, verapamil

Note: Cutaneous side effects of beta-receptor blockaders are clinically polymorphous. They apparently appear after several months of continuous therapy. Atypical psoriasiform, lichen planus-like, and eczematous chronic rashes are mainly observed. (1983): Hödl St, *Z Hautkr* (German) 1:58, 17

Reactions

Skin
- Acne
- Angioedema
- Cold extremities
- Dermatitis (eye-drops) [2]
- Diaphoresis (<1%) [1]
- Edema
- Exanthems
- Exfoliative dermatitis
- Facial edema
- Flushing
- Lupus erythematosus
- Peripheral edema (<1%)
- Photosensitivity
- Pigmentation
- Pruritus
- Psoriasis
- Purpura (<1%)
- Rash (sic) (2.5%)
- Raynaud's phenomenon (<1%)
- Vesiculobullous eruption
- Xerosis

Hair
- Hair – alopecia

Nails
- Nails – discoloration (bluish)

Other
- Anaphylactoid reactions
- Dysgeusia (from topical application)
- Headache
- Myalgia
- Paresthesias (2%)
- Peyronie's disease
- Tinnitus
- Xerostomia

CARVEDILOL

Trade name: Coreg (GSK)
Other common trade names: *Dibloc; Dilatrend; Dimitone; Kredex; Querto*
Indications: Hypertension
Category: Antihypertensive; Beta-adrenoceptor blocker
Half-life: 7–10 hours

Reactions

Skin
- Allergic reactions (sic) (<1%) [1]
- Angioedema [1]
- Diaphoresis (2.9%)
- Edema (generalized) (5.1%)
- Exanthems (<1%) [2]
- Exfoliative dermatitis (<1%)
- Infections (2.2%)
- Peripheral edema (1.4%)
- Photosensitivity (<1%)
- Pruritus (<1%) [1]
- Psoriasis (<1%)
- Purpura (1–10%)
- Rash (sic) (<1%)
- Stevens–Johnson syndrome [1]

Hair
- Hair – alopecia (<0.1%)

Other
- Anaphylactoid reactions (<1%)
- Headache
- Hyperesthesia (<1%)
- Myalgia (3.4%)
- Pain (8.6%)
- Paresthesias (2%)
- Xerostomia (<1%)

CHLOROTHIAZIDE

Trade names: Aldoclor (Merck); Diuril (Merck)
Other common trade names: *Azide; Chlothin; Chlotride; Diurazide; Diuret; Saluretil; Saluric*
Indications: Hypertension, edema
Category: Antihypertensive; Thiazide diuretic
Half-life: 1–2 hours
Clinically important, potentially hazardous interactions with: digoxin, lithium

Reactions

Skin
- Bullous eruption
- Erythema multiforme
- Exanthems [6]
- Exfoliative dermatitis
- Fixed eruption [1]
- Lichenoid eruption [4]
- Lupus erythematosus [1]
- Photosensitivity (<1%) [11]
- Pruritus [3]
- Purpura [6]
- Rash (sic) (<1%)
- Stevens–Johnson syndrome
- Toxic epidermal necrolysis
- Urticaria [1]
- Vasculitis [3]

Hair
- Hair – alopecia

Eyes
- Dyschromatopsia

Other
- Anaphylactoid reactions
- Dysgeusia
- Oral lesions
- Paresthesias (<1%)

***Note:** Chlorothiazide is a sulfonamide and can be absorbed systemically. Sulfonamides can produce severe, possibly fatal, reactions such as toxic epidermal necrolysis and Stevens–Johnson syndrome

CHLORPROPAMIDE

Trade name: Diabinese (Pfizer)
Other common trade names: *Apo-Chlorpropamide; Arodoc C; Chlormide; Diabemide; Diabenese; Insogen; Melormin; Tesmel*
Indications: Diabetes
Category: First generation sulfonylurea
Half-life: 30–42 hours
Clinically important, potentially hazardous interactions with: garlic

Reactions

Skin
- Angioedema [1]
- Bullous eruption (<1%)
- Dermatitis [1]
- Edema (<1%)
- Erythema multiforme (<1%) [7]
- Erythema nodosum (<1%) [2]
- Exanthems (1–5%) [3]

Exfoliative dermatitis [7]
Fixed eruption [1]
Flushing [19]
Granulomas [1]
Lichenoid eruption [4]
Lupus erythematosus [1]
Photosensitivity (1–10%) [3]
Pruritus (<3%) [2]
Purpura [8]
Rash (sic) (1–10%) [1]
Side effects (sic) [3]
Stevens–Johnson syndrome [5]
Toxic epidermal necrolysis [2]
Urticaria (1–10%) [3]
Vasculitis [2]

Hair

Hair – alopecia [1]

Other

Acute intermittent porphyria
Death
Oral lichenoid eruption [3]
Paresthesias
Porphyria [1]
Porphyria cutanea tarda [1]
Tongue ulceration [1]

***Note:** Chlorpropamide is a sulfonamide and can be absorbed systemically. Sulfonamides can produce severe, possibly fatal, reactions such as toxic epidermal necrolysis and Stevens–Johnson syndrome

CHLORTHALIDONE

Trade names: Combipres; Hygroton; Tenoretic (AstraZeneca); Thalitone (Monarch)
Other common trade names: *Higroton; Hydro-Long; Hypertol; Igroton; Thalidone; Uridon*
Indications: Hypertension
Category: Antihypertensive; Thiazide diuretic
Half-life: 35–50 hours
Clinically important, potentially hazardous interactions with: digoxin, lithium

Combipres is chlorthalidone and clonidine

Reactions

Skin

Erythema multiforme
Exanthems
Exfoliative dermatitis
Lupus erythematosus
Necrotizing vasculitis
Photosensitivity (1–10%) [2]
Psoriasis [1]
Purpura (<1%)
Rash (sic) (<1%)
Stevens–Johnson syndrome
Toxic epidermal necrolysis [1]
Urticaria (<1%) [1]
Vasculitis (<1%) [1]

Hair

Hair – alopecia

Eyes

Dyschromatopsia

Other

Headache
Paresthesias (<1%)
Pseudoporphyria [1]

***Note:** Chlorthalidone is a sulfonamide and can be absorbed systemically. Sulfonamides can produce severe, possibly fatal, reactions such as toxic epidermal necrolysis and Stevens–Johnson syndrome

CHOLESTYRAMINE

Trade name: Questran (Par)
Other common trade names: *Chol-Less; Colestrol; Lismol; PMS-Cholestyramine; Prevalite; Quantalan; Questran Lite*
Indications: Pruritus associated with biliary obstruction, primary hypercholesterolemia
Category: Antidiarrheal; Antihyperlipidemic; Antipruritic (cholestasis)
Half-life: N/A
Clinically important, potentially hazardous interactions with: acetaminophen, acitretin, aspirin, chloroquine, cyclosporine, digoxin, doxepin, hydroxychloroquine, isotretinoin, lovastatin, mycophenolate, raloxifene, sulfasalazine, tetracycline, valproic acid

Reactions

Skin
- Edema
- Exanthems
- Rash (sic) (<1%)
- Urticaria

Hematopoietic
- Ecchymoses

Other
- Dysgeusia
- Osteomalacia [1]
- Paresthesias
- Tinnitus
- Tongue irritation (<1%)

CILOSTAZOL

Synonym: OPC13013
Trade name: Pletal (Pfizer)
Indications: Peripheral vascular disease, intermittent claudication
Category: Platelet aggregation inhibitor
Half-life: 11–13 hours
Clinically important, potentially hazardous interactions with: clarithromycin, erythromycin, fondaparinux

Reactions

Skin
- Chills (<2%)
- Edema (<2%)
- Facial edema (<2%)
- Furunculosis (<2%)
- Hypertrophy
- Infections
- Peripheral edema (7–9%)
- Pruritus
- Purpura (<2%)
- Rash (sic) (2%)
- Urticaria (<2%)
- Xerosis (<2%)

Hematopoietic
- Ecchymoses (<2%)

Other
- Headache
- Hyperesthesia (2%)
- Myalgia (2–3%)
- Paresthesias (2%)
- Tongue edema (<2%)
- Vaginitis (<2%)

CLOFIBRATE

Other common trade names: *Abitrate; Claripex; Col; Lipavlon; Novo-Fibrate; Regelan N; Skleromexe*
Indications: Type III hyperlipidemia
Category: Antihyperlipidemic
Half-life: 6–25 hours after a single dose
Clinically important, potentially hazardous interactions with: anisindione, dicumarol, warfarin

Reactions

Skin
- Dermatitis [3]
- Diaphoresis
- Erythema multiforme [1]
- Exanthems [6]
- Exfoliative dermatitis [1]
- Facial rash [1]
- Lupus erythematosus [1]
- Photosensitivity [4]
- Pruritus (<1%)
- Purpura [1]
- Rash (sic) (<1%)
- Sarcoidosis [1]
- Stevens–Johnson syndrome [1]
- Toxic epidermal necrolysis
- Urticaria (<1%)
- Vesiculobullous eruption [1]
- Xerosis

Hair
- Hair – alopecia (<1%) [1]
- Hair – dry (<1%)

Other
- Dysgeusia
- Gynecomastia
- Hypogeusia
- Myalgia (<1%) [3]
- Oral ulceration [1]
- Rhabdomyolysis [1]
- Stomatitis

CLONIDINE

Trade names: Catapres (Boehringer Ingelheim); Combivent (Boehringer Ingelheim)
Other common trade names: *Barclyd; Catapresan; Daipres; Dixarit; Duraclon; Haemiton; Nu-Clonidine; Sulmidine*
Indications: Hypertension
Category: Alpha-2-adrenoceptor blocker; Antihypertensive
Half-life: 6–24 hours
Clinically important, potentially hazardous interactions with: acebutolol, amitriptyline, amoxapine, atenolol, betaxolol, carteolol, clomipramine, desipramine, doxepin, esmolol, imipramine, metoprolol, nadolol, nortriptyline, penbutolol, pindolol, propranolol, protriptyline, timolol, trimipramine, verapamil

Combipres is clonidine and chlorthalidone

Reactions

Skin
- Angioedema (<1%) [1]
- Depigmentation [2]
- Dermatitis (from patch) (20%) [23]
- Diaphoresis [1]
- Eczema [2]
- Edema
- Erythema [2]
- Exanthems
- Excoriations [1]
- Herpes simplex [1]
- Irritation (from patch) [1]
- Lupus erythematosus [4]
- Pemphigus (anogenital and cicatricial) [1]
- Peripheral edema
- Pigmentation [2]
- Pityriasis rosea [2]
- Pruritus (>5%) [5]
- Psoriasis [1]
- Rash (sic) (1–10%) [1]
- Raynaud's phenomenon (<1%)
- Scaling [1]
- Ulcerations (1–10%)
- Urticaria (<1%)
- Vesiculation [1]

Hair
- Hair – alopecia (<1%)

Other
- Acute intermittent porphyria
- Application-site vesicles [1]
- Dysgeusia (from patch)
- Gynecomastia (<1%)
- Headache
- Hyperesthesia (1–10%)
- Immune complex disease [1]
- Induration [1]
- Pseudolymphoma [1]
- Seizures [1]
- Xerostomia (40%) [7]

CLOPIDOGREL

Trade name: Plavix (Bristol-Myers Squibb) (Sanofi-Aventis)
Indications: Atherosclerotic events
Category: Antiplatelet (thienopyridine derivative)
Half-life: ~8 hours
Clinically important, potentially hazardous interactions with: anisindione, dicumarol, fondaparinux, warfarin

Reactions

Skin
- Allergic reactions (sic) (1–2.5%)
- Angioedema [1]
- Bullous eruption (1–2.5%)
- Cellulitis [1]
- Eczema (1–2.5%)
- Edema (3–5%)
- Exanthems (1–2.5%) [2]
- Flu-like syndrome (7.5%)
- Lichenoid eruption (photosensitive) [1]
- Photosensitivity (lichenoid) [1]
- Pruritus (3.3%) [1]
- Purpura (5.3%) [8]
- Rash (sic) (4.2%)
- Toxic dermatitis [1]
- Ulcerations (1–2.5%)
- Urticaria (1–2.5%) [1]

Eyes
- Ocular hemorrhage [1]

Hematopoietic
Ecchymoses [1]
Neutropenia [1]
Thrombocytopenic purpura [10]

Other
Ageusia [1]
Fever [1]
Headache
Hyperesthesia (1–2.5%)
Hypersensitivity [1]
Paresthesias (1–2.5%)
Rhabdomyolysis [1]

COLESEVELAM

Trade name: Welchol (Sankyo)
Indications: Hypercholesterolemia
Category: Antilipemic; Bile acid sequestrant
Half-life: N/A

Reactions

Skin
Flu-like syndrome

Other
Myalgia (2%)
Oral ulceration

COLESTIPOL

Trade name: Colestid (Pfizer)
Other common trade names: *Cholestabyl; Lestid*
Indications: Primary hypercholesterolemia
Category: Antilipidemic
Half-life: N/A

Reactions

Skin
Dermatitis (<1%)
Edema
Exanthems (<1%)
Urticaria (<1%)

CYCLOTHIAZIDE

Trade name: Anhydron
Other common trade names: *Doburil; Valmiran*
Indications: Edema, hypertension
Category: Thiazide diuretic
Half-life: N/A
Clinically important, potentially hazardous interactions with: digoxin

Reactions

Skin
- Exanthems (<1%)
- Photosensitivity
- Purpura
- Rash (sic)
- Urticaria
- Vasculitis

Other
- Paresthesias

***Note:** Cyclothiazide is a sulfonamide and can be absorbed systemically. Sulfonamides can produce severe, possibly fatal, reactions such as toxic epidermal necrolysis and Stevens–Johnson syndrome

DALTEPARIN

Trade name: Fragmin (Pfizer)
Other common trade name: *Fragmine*
Indications: Prophylaxis of deep vein thrombosis
Category: Anticoagulant; Low-molecular weight heparin
Half-life: 4–8 hours
Clinically important, potentially hazardous interactions with: butabarbital, danaparoid

Reactions

Skin
- Allergic reactions (sic) (1–10%) [3]
- Bullous eruption (1–10%) [1]
- Exanthems (<1%)
- Lesions [1]
- Necrosis
- Pruritus (1–10%)
- Rash (sic) (1–10%)

Hair
- Hair – alopecia [2]

Other
- Anaphylactoid reactions (1–10%) [1]
- Injection-site edema [1]
- Injection-site hematoma (1–10%)
- Injection-site pain (1–10%)
- Injection-site pruritus [1]

DANAPAROID

Trade name: Orgaran (Organon)
Indications: Prevention of postoperative deep thrombosis
Category: Anticoagulant
Half-life: ~24 hours
Clinically important, potentially hazardous interactions with: butabarbital, dalteparin, enoxaparin, heparin

Reactions

Skin
- Allergic reactions (sic) (<1%) [1]
- Edema (2.6%)
- Infections (2.1%)
- Peripheral edema (3.3%)
- Pruritus (3.9%)
- Purpura
- Rash (sic) (2.1–4.8%) [1]

Other
- Injection-site hematoma (5%)
- Injection-site infiltrated plaques [3]
- Injection-site pain (7.6–13.7%)
- Injection-site reactions [1]
- Paresthesias

DEXMEDETOMIDINE

Trade name: Precedex (Abbott)
Indications: Sedation for intensive care unit intubation
Category: Alpha-adrenoceptor blocker; Sedative
Half-life: 2 hours

Reactions

Skin
- Diaphoresis (<1%)
- Infections (2%)
- Xerosis

Eyes
- Photopsia (<1%)

Other
- Pain (3%)
- Sialopenia [1]

DIAZOXIDE

Trade name: Hyperstat (Schering)
Other common trade names: *Eudimine; Proglicem; Proglycem; Sefulken*
Indications: Hypoglycemia, hypertension
Category: Antihypertensive; Antihypoglycemic
Half-life: 20–36 hours
Clinically important, potentially hazardous interactions with: phenytoin

Reactions

Skin
- Candidiasis
- Cellulitis (<1%)
- Diaphoresis
- Edema
- Exanthems
- Flushing (<1%)
- Herpes
- Leukomelanosis [1]
- Lichenoid eruption [2]
- Photosensitivity [1]
- Pruritus
- Purpura
- Rash (sic) (<1%)

Urticaria
Xerosis [1]

Hair
Hair – alopecia [2]
Hair – hypertrichosis (<1%) [10]

Other
Ageusia
Dysgeusia
Headache
Hypersensitivity
Injection-site pain (<1%)
Injection-site phlebitis (<1%)
Paresthesias
Sialorrhea
Tinnitus
Xerostomia

DICUMAROL

Synonym: bishydroxycoumarin
Trade name: Dicumarol
Other common trade names: *Apekumarol; Dicumol; Embolin*
Indications: Atrial fibrillation, pulmonary embolism, venous thrombosis
Category: Anticoagulant
Half-life: 1–4 days
Clinically important, potentially hazardous interactions with: allopurinol, amiodarone, amobarbital, aprobarbital, aspirin, bivalirudin, butabarbital, butalbital, cimetidine, clofibrate, clopidogrel, cyclosporine, delavirdine, disulfiram, fenofibrate, fluconazole, gemfibrozil, imatinib, itraconazole, ketoconazole, levothyroxine, liothyronine, mephobarbital, methimazole, metronidazole, miconazole, penicillins, pentobarbital, phenobarbital, piperacillin, primidone, propylthiouracil, quinidine, quinine, rifabutin, rifampin, rifapentine, rofecoxib, secobarbital, sulfinpyrazone, testosterone, zileuton

Reactions

Skin
Acral purpura [1]
Angioedema (<1%)
Bullous eruption [1]
Dermatitis [2]
Exanthems [5]
Hemorrhage [3]
Necrosis [10]
Pigmentation [1]
Pruritus (<1%)
Purplish erythema (feet and toes) [2]
Purpura [2]
Rash (sic)
Urticaria [3]
Vesiculation [1]

Hair
Hair – alopecia (1–10%) [5]

Hematopoietic
Ecchymoses [1]

Other
Hypersensitivity
Oral ulceration
Priapism

DIGOXIN

Trade name: Lanoxin (GSK)
Other common trade names: *Cardigox; Digacin; Digoxine; Eudigox; Lanicor; Lenoxin; Novo-Digoxin*
Indications: Congestive heart failure, atrial fibrillation
Category: Antiarrhythmic; Cardiac glycoside; Inotropic
Half-life: 36–48 hours
Clinically important, potentially hazardous interactions with: alprazolam, amiodarone, amphotericin B, arbutamine, bendroflumethiazide, benzthiazide, bumetanide, chlorothiazide, chlorthalidone, cholestyramine, clarithromycin, cyclosporine, cyclothiazide, demeclocycline, **devil's claw**, doxycycline, erythromycin, esomeprazole, ethacrynic acid, furosemide, **ginseng**, **hawthorn fruit, leaf, flower extract**, hydrochlorothiazide, hydroflumethiazide, indapamide, **licorice**, mepenzolate, methyclothiazide, metolazone, minocycline, **mistletoe**, oxytetracycline, polythiazide, propafenone, propantheline, quinethazone, quinidine, rifampin, **sarsaparilla**, **senna**, **siberian ginseng**, **st john's wort**, telithromycin, teriparatide, tetracycline, trichlormethiazide, verapamil

Reactions

Skin
Angioedema
Bullous eruption [1]
Diaphoresis [1]
Exanthems (1.6%) [3]
Pruritus [1]
Psoriasis [1]
Purpura [1]
Rash (sic)
Urticaria [2]
Vasculitis [1]

Hair
Hair – alopecia

Nails
Nails – loss (finger- and toenails)

Eyes
Dyschromatopsia (green) [1]

Other
Gynecomastia [1]
Headache

DILTIAZEM

Trade names: Cardizem (Biovail); Cartia-XT; Dilacor XR (Watson); Diltia-XT; Teczem (Sanofi-Aventis); Tiazac (Forest)
Other common trade names: *Alti-Diltiazem; Britiazem; Calcicard; Deltazen; Dilrene; Diltahexal; Nu-Diltiaz; Presoken; Tiamate; Tilazem; Tildiem*
Indications: Angina, essential hypertension
Category: Antianginal; Antiarrhythmic; Calcium channel blocker
Half-life: 5–8 hours (for extended-release capsules)
Clinically important, potentially hazardous interactions with: alfuzosin, amiodarone, aprepitant, carbamazepine, corticosteroids, cyclosporine, epirubicin, erythromycin, **mistletoe**, simvastatin

Teczem is diltiazem and enalapril

Reactions

Skin
- Acne [1]
- Acute generalized exanthematous pustulosis (AGEP) [12]
- Adverse effects (sic) [1]
- Angioedema [2]
- Capillaritis (Schamberg's) [1]
- Dermatitis
- Diaphoresis [2]
- Edema (1–10%) [4]
- Erythema [2]
- Erythema multiforme (1–31%) [9]
- Exanthems [16]
- Exfoliative dermatitis (<1%) [6]
- Flushing (1–10%) [5]
- Hyperkeratosis (feet) [1]
- Lichenoid eruption (photosensitive) [2]
- Lupus erythematosus [5]
- Palmar–plantar desquamation [1]
- Peripheral edema (5–8%) [2]
- Petechiae (<1%)
- Photosensitivity (<1%) [11]
- Pigmentation [4]
- Pruritus (<1%) [7]
- Psoriasis [3]
- Purpura (<1%) [3]
- Pustular psoriasis [1]
- Pustules [2]
- Rash (sic) (1.3%) [3]
- Side effects (sic) [2]
- Stevens–Johnson syndrome [4]
- Subcorneal pustular dermatosis [2]
- Thickening [2]
- Toxic dermatitis [1]
- Toxic epidermal necrolysis [4]
- Toxic erythema [2]
- Ulcerations of legs [2]
- Urticaria (<1%) [4]
- Vasculitis (<1%) [6]

Hair
- Hair – alopecia (<1%) [2]
- Hair – hirsutism [1]

Nails
- Nails – dystrophy [1]

Eyes
- Periorbital edema [1]

Hematopoietic
- Ecchymoses (<1%)

Other
- Dysgeusia (<1%) [1]
- Erythromelalgia [1]
- Fever [1]
- Gingival hypertrophy (21%) [6]
- Gynecomastia [1]
- Headache
- Hypersensitivity [1]
- Lymphadenopathy [1]
- Myoclonus [1]
- Parageusia (<1%)
- Paresthesias (<1%) [1]
- Parkinsonism [2]
- Pseudolymphoma [1]
- Rhabdomyolysis [3]
- Tinnitus
- Tremor (<1%)
- Xerostomia (<1%) [2]

DIPYRIDAMOLE

Trade names: Aggrenox (Boehringer Ingelheim); Persantine (Boehringer Ingelheim)
Other common trade names: *Cardoxin; Cleridium; Coronarine; Coroxin; Curantyl N; Dipridacot; Lodimol; Novo-Dipiradol; Persantin*
Indications: Thromboembolic complications following cardiac valve replacement
Category: Platelet aggregation inhibitor
Half-life: 10–12 hours
Clinically important, potentially hazardous interactions with: adenosine, **dong quai**, fondaparinux, reteplase

Aggrenox is dipyridamole and aspirin

Reactions

Skin
Allergic reactions (sic) (<1%)
Angioedema [1]
Diaphoresis (0.4%)
Edema (0.3%)
Erythema multiforme
Exanthems [1]
Flushing (3.4%)
Pruritus [1]
Psoriasis [1]
Purpura (1.4%) [1]
Rash (sic) (2.3%) [1]
Stevens–Johnson syndrome [1]
Toxic epidermal necrolysis [1]
Ulcerations (<1%)
Urticaria [1]

Other
Anaphylactoid reactions [1]
Dysgeusia (0.1%)
Gingivitis (<1%)
Headache
Hyperesthesia (0.5%)
Injection-site pain (0.1%)
Injection-site reactions (sic) (0.4%)
Mastodynia (0.03%)
Myalgia (0.9%)
Paresthesias (1.3%)
Pseudopolymyalgia [1]
Tremor (<1%)

DISOPYRAMIDE

Trade name: Norpace (Pfizer)
Other common trade names: *Dimodan; Dirythmin SA; Disonorm; Durbis; Isorythm*
Indications: Ventricular arrhythmias
Category: Antiarrhythmic
Half-life: 4–10 hours
Clinically important, potentially hazardous interactions with: arsenic, ciprofloxacin, clarithromycin, enoxacin, erythromycin, gatifloxacin, lomefloxacin, moxifloxacin, norfloxacin, ofloxacin, sparfloxacin

Reactions

Skin
Angioedema
Dermatitis
Edema (1–3%)

Erythema nodosum [1]
Exanthems (1–5%) [1]
Lupus erythematosus (<1%) [2]
Photosensitivity [1]
Pruritus (1–3%)
Purpura [1]
Rash (sic) (generalized) (1–3%)
Urticaria
Xerosis

Hair

Hair – alopecia

Other

Gynecomastia (<1%)
Headache
Oral lesions (40%) [1]
Paresthesias (<1%)
Torsades de pointes [1]
Xerostomia (32%) [1]

DOBUTAMINE

Trade name: Dobutrex (Lilly)
Other common trade names: *Cardiject; Dobril; Dobuject; Dobutamin; Inotrex; Oxiken; Tobrex*
Indications: Cardiac surgery, heart failure
Category: Adrenergic agonist; Inotropic sympathomimetic; Vasopressor
Half-life: 2 minutes
Clinically important, potentially hazardous interactions with: furazolidone

Reactions

Skin

Cellulitis [1]
Erythema [1]
Necrosis [1]
Pruritus [2]

Other

Headache
Hypersensitivity [1]
Injection-site pain
Injection-site phlebitis
Paresthesias (1–10%)
Phlebitis

DOFETILIDE

Trade name: Tikosyn (Pfizer)
Indications: Conversion of atrial fibrillation and atrial flutter to normal sinus rhythm
Category: Class III antiarrhythmic
Half-life: 10 hours
Clinically important, potentially hazardous interactions with: atazanavir, chlorpromazine, cimetidine, co Trimoxazole, fluphenazine, ketoconazole, medroxyprogesterone, mesoridazine, prochlorperazine, progestins, promethazine, thioridazine, trifluoperazine, trimethoprim, verapamil

Reactions

Skin
- Angioedema (<2%)
- Diaphoresis (>2%)
- Edema
- Flu-like syndrome (4%)
- Peripheral edema (>2%)
- Rash (sic) (3%)

Other
- Headache
- Paresthesias (<2%)
- Torsades de pointes [2]

DOPAMINE

Trade names: Dopastat; Intropin
Other common trade names: *Cardiosteril; Dopamin; Dopamin AWD; Dynatra; Revimine*
Indications: Hemodynamic imbalances present in shock
Category: Adrenergic agonist; Inotropic sympathomimetic; Vasopressor
Half-life: 2 minutes
Clinically important, potentially hazardous interactions with: ethotoin, fosphenytoin, furazolidone, mephenytoin, phenelzine, phenytoin, tranylcypromine

Reactions

Skin
- Exanthems
- Necrosis [1]
- Piloerection
- Pruritus
- Raynaud's phenomenon (<1%)
- Urticaria

Hair
- Hair – alopecia

Other
- Headache
- Injection-site extravasation [2]
- Injection-site gangrene [1]
- Injection-site necrosis (<1%) [3]
- Injection-site piloerection and vasoconstriction [1]
- Peripheral ischemia [1]
- Symmetric peripheral gangrene [1]

DOXAZOSIN

Trade name: Cardura (Pfizer)
Other common trade names: *Alfadil; Cardoxan; Cardular; Dedralen; Diblocin; Supressin*
Indications: Hypertension
Category: Alpha-adrenoceptor blocker; Antihypertensive
Half-life: 19–22 hours
Clinically important, potentially hazardous interactions with: tadalafil, vardenafil

Reactions

Skin
- Bruising [1]
- Diaphoresis (1.4%) [1]
- Eczema (<0.5%)

Edema (4%)
Exanthems (1.7%) [1]
Facial edema (1%)
Flu-like syndrome (1.1%)
Flushing (1%) [1]
Hot flashes (<1%)
Lichen planus [1]
Lichenoid eruption [1]
Lupus erythematosus [1]
Pallor (<1%)
Peripheral edema
Pruritus (1%)
Purpura (<0.5%)
Rash (sic) (1%) [1]
Urticaria [1]
Xerosis (<0.5%)

Hair

Hair – alopecia (<0.5%) [1]
Hair – hypertrichosis [1]

Other

Dysgeusia (<0.5%) [1]
Headache
Hyperesthesia (<1%)
Mastodynia (<1%)
Myalgia (1%)
Paresthesias
Parosmia (<0.05%)
Tinnitus
Xerostomia (2%) [1]

EDROPHONIUM

Trade names: Enlon (Baxter); Tensilon (Valeant)
Indications: Myasthenia gravis diagnosis
Category: Anticholinesterase; Antidote; Neuromuscular blocker
Half-life: 1.8 hours
Clinically important, potentially hazardous interactions with: corticosteroids, galantamine

Reactions

Skin

Diaphoresis (>10%)
Flushing
Rash (sic)
Urticaria

Other

Anaphylactoid reactions
Headache
Hypersensitivity (<1%)
Sialorrhea (>10%)
Thrombophlebitis (<1%)

ENALAPRIL

Trade names: Lexxel (AstraZeneca); Teczem (Sanofi-Aventis); Vasotec (Biovail)
Other common trade names: *Amprace; Apo-Enalapril; Enaladil; Enapren; Glioten; Innovace; Pres; Renitec; Reniten; Xanef*
Indications: Hypertension
Category: Angiotensin-converting enzyme (ACE) inhibitor; Antihypertensive
Half-life: 11 hours
Clinically important, potentially hazardous interactions with: amiloride, spironolactone, triamterene

Lexxel is enalapril and felodipine; Teczem is enalapril and diltiazem; Vaseretic is enalapril and hydrochlorothiazide

Reactions

Skin
- Acantholysis [1]
- Angioedema (<1%) [62]
- Bullous pemphigoid [2]
- Diaphoresis (<1%) [1]
- Erythema [1]
- Erythema multiforme (<1%)
- Exanthems (1%) [9]
- Exfoliative dermatitis (<1%)
- Flushing (<1%) [2]
- Herpes zoster (<1%)
- Lichenoid eruption [2]
- Lupus erythematosus [1]
- Mycosis fungoides [1]
- Pemphigus [8]
- Pemphigus foliaceus [2]
- Pemphigus vegetans [1]
- Photosensitivity (<1%) [3]
- Pruritus (<1%) [4]
- Psoriasis [2]
- Purpura [1]
- Rash (sic) (1.4%) [5]
- Stevens–Johnson syndrome (<1%)
- Toxic epidermal necrolysis (<1%)
- Toxic pustuloderma [1]
- Urticaria (<1%) [5]
- Vasculitis (<1%) [2]

Hair
- Hair – alopecia (<1%) [1]

Nails
- Nails – dystrophy [1]

Other
- Ageusia [3]
- Anaphylactoid reactions (<1%) [1]
- Anosmia (<1%)
- Cough (8–23%) [8]
- Death [1]
- Dysesthesia (<1%)
- Dysgeusia (1–10%) [5]
- Glossitis (<1%)
- Glossopyrosis [1]
- Gynecomastia [1]
- Headache
- Myalgia (<1%)
- Oral bleeding [1]
- Oral burn [1]
- Oral lesions (<0.5%) [4]
- Oral mucosal lichenoid eruption [1]
- Oral ulceration [2]
- Paresthesias (<1%)
- Pseudopolymyalgia [2]
- Stomatitis (<1%)
- Tinnitus
- Tongue edema [3]
- Xerostomia (<1%)

ENOXAPARIN

Trade name: Lovenox (Sanofi-Aventis)
Other common trade names: *Clexan; Clexane 40; Klexane*
Indications: Prevention of deep vein thrombosis
Category: Anticoagulant ; Low-molecular weight heparin
Half-life: 4.5 hours
Clinically important, potentially hazardous interactions with: butabarbital, danaparoid

Reactions

Skin

Angioedema [1]
Edema (3%)
Erythema (1–10%) [1]
Erythema multiforme [1]
Exanthems [3]
Hematomas [1]
Necrosis (<1%) [2]
Peripheral edema (3%)
Pruritus [2]
Purpura (1–10%)
Side effects (sic) (0.2%) [1]
Urticaria [2]
Vesiculation (<1%)

Hematopoietic

Ecchymoses (2%)

Other

Anaphylactoid reactions (<1%) [1]
Anxiety [1]
Cough [1]
Hypersensitivity [5]
Injection-site erythema [1]
Injection-site exanthems [1]
Injection-site hematoma [1]
Injection-site infiltrated plaques [2]
Injection-site necrosis [3]
Injection-site pain [1]
Injection-site pruritus [1]

EPHEDRA

Scientific names: *Ephedra equisetina; Ephedra intermedia; Ephedra sinica; Ephedra vulgaris*
Family: Gnetaceae
Trade and other common names: Joint Fir; Ma Huang; Popotillo; Sea Grape; Teamster's Tea; Yellow Astringent; Yellow Horse
Category: Cardiovascular stimulant; CNS stimulant
Purported indications and other uses: Bronchospasm, asthma, bronchitis, allergy, appetite suppressant, colds, flu, fever, chills, edema, headache, anhidrosis, diuretic, joint and bone pain
Half-life: N/A
Clinically important, potentially hazardous interactions with: acetazolamide, amitriptyline, **caffeine**, ephedrine, epinephrine, guanethidine, **guarana**, olmesartan, phenelzine, phenylpropanolamine, selegiline, sibutramine

Reactions

Skin

Adverse effects (sic) [3]
Flushing

Other

Death [3]
Eosinophilia–myalgia syndrome [1]
Hypersensitivity
Seizures [3]
Side effects (sic) [1]
Tremor
Xerostomia [1]

Note: The FDA has recently banned Ephedra because of serious side effects

EPHEDRINE

Trade names: Ectasule; Efedron; Ephedsol; Marax; Pretz-D; Rynatuss (MedPointe); Vicks Vatronol (Procter & Gamble)
Indications: Nasal congestion, acute hypotensive states, asthma
Category: Adrenergic agonist; Sympathomimetic bronchodilator
Half-life: 3–6 hours
Clinically important, potentially hazardous interactions with: ephedra, furazolidone, guanethidine, **guarana**, methyldopa, phenelzine, phenylpropanolamine, selegiline, tranylcypromine

Reactions

Skin
Bullous eruption [1]
Dermatitis (following topical application) [3]
Dermatitis [2]
Diaphoresis (1–10%)
Edema
Exanthems [1]
Exfoliative dermatitis [1]
Fixed eruption [6]
Pallor (1–10%)
Purpura [1]
Toxic epidermal necrolysis [1]
Urticaria [2]
Vasculitis [1]

Other
Death [1]
Headache
Myalgia [1]
Seizures [1]
Trembling (1–10%)
Tremor (1–10%) [1]
Xerostomia (1–10%)

EPINEPHRINE

Synonym: adrenaline
Trade names: Adrenalin (Monarch); AsthmaHaler; Bronitin; Bronkaid; Epifrin; Epipen (DEY); MedihalerEpi; Primatene
Other common trade names: *Adrenaline; Ana-Guard; Epi E-Z Pen; Eppy; Eppystabil; Isopto-Epinal; Primatene Mist; S-2; Simplene*
Indications: Cardiac arrest, hay fever, asthma, anaphylaxis
Category: Adrenergic agonist; Sympathomimetic bronchodilator
Duration of action: 1–4 hours
Clinically important, potentially hazardous interactions with: albuterol, amitriptyline, amoxapine, atenolol, carteolol, chlorpromazine, clomipramine, cocaine, desipramine, doxepin, **ephedra**, furazolidone, halothane, imipramine, metoprolol, nadolol, nortriptyline, penbutolol, phenelzine, phenoxybenzamine, phenylephrine, pindolol, prazosin, propranolol, protriptyline, terbutaline, thioridazine, timolol, tranylcypromine, trimipramine

Reactions

Skin
- Dermatitis [4]
- Diaphoresis (1–10%)
- Exanthems
- Fixed eruption
- Flushing (1–10%)
- Necrosis [1]
- Pallor (<1%)
- Pemphigus (cicatricial) [2]
- Urticaria

Hair
- Hair – alopecia [1]

Other
- Headache
- Injection-site necrosis
- Injection-site pain
- Injection-site urticaria
- Trembling (1–10%)
- Xerostomia (<1%)

EPLERENONE

Trade name: Inspra (Pfizer)
Indications: Hypertension
Category: Antihypertensive; Selective aldosterone blocker
Half-life: 4–6 hours
Clinically important, potentially hazardous interactions with: erythromycin, fluconazole, itraconazole, ketoconazole, saquinavir, **st john's wort**, verapamil

Reactions

Skin
- Flu-like syndrome (2%)

Other
- Cough (2%)
- Dizziness (3%)
- Fatigue (2%)
- Gynecomastia (males <1%)
- Headache
- Mastodynia (males <1%)

EPROSARTAN

Trade name: Teveten (Biovail)
Indications: Hypertension
Category: Angiotensin II receptor antagonist; Antihypertensive
Half-life: 5–9 hours

Reactions

Skin
- Angioedema
- Diaphoresis (<1%)
- Eczema (<1%)
- Exanthems (<1%)
- Facial edema (<1%)
- Furunculosis (<1%)
- Herpes simplex (<1%)
- Hot flashes (<1%)
- Peripheral edema (<1%)

Pruritus (<1%)
Purpura (<1%)
Rash (sic) (<1%)

Other
Burning mouth syndrome [1]
Cough (5%) [1]
Dysgeusia [1]
Gingivitis (<1%)
Myalgia
Paresthesias (<1%)
Tendinitis (<1%)
Tremor (<1%)
Xerostomia (<1%)

EPTIFIBATIDE

Trade name: Integrilin (Millennium) (Schering)
Indications: Acute coronary syndrome, unstable angina
Category: Antiplatelet; Platelet aggregation inhibitor
Half-life: 2.5 hours
Clinically important, potentially hazardous interactions with: fondaparinux

Reactions

Other
Anaphylactoid reactions (<1%)
Injection-site reactions (sic)

ESMOLOL

Trade name: Brevibloc (Baxter)
Indications: Tachyarrhythmias, tachycardia
Category: Antiarrhythmic class II; Antihypertensive; Beta-adrenoceptor blocker
Half-life: 9 minutes
Clinically important, potentially hazardous interactions with: clonidine, verapamil

Reactions

Skin
Acne (<1%)
Cold extremities
Diaphoresis (>10%)
Eczema (<1%)
Edema (<1%)
Erythema (<1%)
Exfoliative dermatitis (<1%)
Facial edema
Flushing (<1%)
Necrosis (<1%)
Pallor (<1%)
Pigmentation (<1%)
Psoriasis (<1%)
Purpura
Rash (sic)
Urticaria

Hair
Hair – alopecia

Other
Dysgeusia
Injection-site inflammation [1]
Injection-site pain (8%)
Injection-site reactions (sic) (1–10%)
Paresthesias (<1%)
Thrombophlebitis (<1%)
Xerostomia (<1%)

ETHACRYNIC ACID

Trade name: Edecrin (Merck)
Other common trade names: *Edecril; Edecrina; Hydromedin; Reomax*
Indications: Edema
Category: Loop diuretic
Half-life: 2–4 hours
Clinically important, potentially hazardous interactions with: amikacin, digoxin, gentamicin, kanamycin, neomycin, streptomycin, tobramycin

Reactions

Skin

Allergic reactions (sic)
Chills (<1%)
Exanthems [1]
Photosensitivity
Purpura (<1%)
Rash (sic) (<1%)
Urticaria
Vasculitis [2]

Other

Injection-site pain
Thrombophlebitis (<1%)
Tinnitus
Xerostomia

EZETIMIBE

Trade name: Zetia
Indications: Hypercholesterolemia
Category: Selective cholesterol-absorption inhibitor
Half-life: 22 hours
Clinically important, potentially hazardous interactions with: cyclosporine, fenofibrate, gemfibrozil

Reactions

Skin

Viral infections (2.2%)

Hair

Hair – loss [1]

Other

Abdominal pain (2.2%)
Arthralgia (3.8%)
Back pain (4.1%) [1]
Cough (2.3%)
Myalgia (5%) [1]

FELODIPINE

Trade names: Lexxel (AstraZeneca); Plendil (AstraZeneca)
Other common trade names: *AGON SR; Hydac; Modip; Munobal; Penedil; Renedil; Splendil*
Indications: Hypertension
Category: Antihypertensive; Calcium channel blocker
Half-life: 11–16 hours
Clinically important, potentially hazardous interactions with: carbamazepine, epirubicin, **grapefruit Juice**, imatinib, telithromycin

Lexxel is enalapril and felodipine

Reactions

Skin
- Diaphoresis [1]
- Edema [1]
- Erythema (1.5%)
- Exanthems [2]
- Facial edema (1.5%)
- Flu-like syndrome (<1%)
- Flushing (>25%) [10]
- Peripheral edema (22%) [5]
- Pruritus (<1%)
- Purpura [1]
- Rash (sic) (1.5%)
- Telangiectasia [2]
- Urticaria (1.5%)

Nails
- Nails – brittle (44%) [1]

Other
- Gingival hypertrophy (2–10%) [1]
- Gynecomastia (<1%)
- Headache
- Myalgia (1.5%)
- Paresthesias (2.5%)
- Tinnitus
- Xerostomia (<1%) [1]

FENOFIBRATE

Synonyms: procetofene; proctofene
Trade name: Tricor (Abbott)
Other common trade name: *Apo-Fenofibrate*
Indications: Hyperlipidemia
Category: Fibric acid cholesterol-lowering agent
Half-life: 20 hours
Clinically important, potentially hazardous interactions with: dicumarol, ezetimibe, lovastatin, warfarin

Reactions

Skin
- Adverse effects (sic) (1–10%) [1]
- Exanthems [1]
- Photosensitivity [10]
- Phototoxicity [2]
- Pruritus (4%)
- Rash (sic) (2–8%) [3]
- Toxic epidermal necrolysis [1]
- Urticaria

Hair

Hair – alopecia [1]

Other

Headache
Muscle tenderness [1]
Muscle toxicity (sic) [2]
Myalgia (<1%) [2]
Myositis [1]
Paresthesias
Polymyositis [1]
Rhabdomyolysis [2]
Septic–toxic shock [1]
Vaginitis

FENOLDOPAM

Trade name: Corlopam (Abbott) (Neurex)
Indications: Hypertension (severe), hypertensive emergency
Category: Peripheral vasodilator
Half-life: ~5 minutes

Reactions

Skin

Diaphoresis
Flushing

Other

Back pain
Chest pain
Dizziness
Headache
Injection-site reactions

FLECAINIDE

Trade name: Tambocor (3M)
Other common trade names: *Almarytm; Apocard; Corflene; Flecaine; Tabco*
Indications: Atrial fibrillation
Category: Antiarrhythmic
Half-life: 7–22 hours
Clinically important, potentially hazardous interactions with: fosamprenavir, ritonavir

Reactions

Skin

Diaphoresis (<3%)
Edema (3.5%)
Exanthems (>1%) [2]
Exfoliative dermatitis (<1%)
Flushing (<3%)
Pruritus (<1%) [1]
Psoriasis [2]
Rash (sic) (<3%)
Urticaria (<1%)

Hair

Hair – alopecia (<1%)

Other

Dysgeusia (<1%) (metallic taste)
Headache
Hyperesthesia (1–10%)
Myalgia (<1%)
Oral edema
Paresthesias (<1%)
Tinnitus

Tongue edema (<1%)
Tremor (5%)
Xerostomia (<1%)

FLUVASTATIN

Trade name: Lescol (Novartis)
Other common trade names: *Cranoc; Locol*
Indications: Hypercholesterolemia
Category: Antihyperlipidemic; HMG-CoA reductase inhibitor
Half-life: 1.2 hours
Clinically important, potentially hazardous interactions with: azithromycin, bosentan, clarithromycin, cyclosporine, erythromycin, gemfibrozil, imatinib

Reactions

Skin
Allergic reactions (sic) (2.6%)
Angioedema
Discoloration
Erythema multiforme
Flu-like syndrome
Flushing
Lupus erythematosus [1]
Photosensitivity
Pruritus
Purpura
Rash (sic) (2.7%) [1]
Stevens–Johnson syndrome
Toxic epidermal necrolysis
Upper respiratory infection (16%)
Urticaria
Vasculitis
Xerosis

Hair
Hair – alopecia [1]
Hair – changes (sic)

Nails
Nails – changes (sic)

Other
Anaphylactoid reactions
Death
Dysgeusia
Gynecomastia
Headache
Myalgia [2]
Myositis [2]
Paresthesias
Rhabdomyolysis [7]

FORMOTEROL

Synonym: Formoterol fumarate
Other common trade name: *Oxeze*
Indications: Asthma, bronchospasm
Category: Beta-2-adrenergic agonist
Half-life: 10–14 hours
Clinically important, potentially hazardous interactions with: clomipramine, desipramine, doxepin, imipramine, nortriptyline, protriptyline, trimipramine

Reactions

Skin
- Angioedema
- Erythema
- Infections (3%)
- Pruritus
- Rash (sic) (1.1%)
- Urticaria
- Viral infections (17.2%)

Other
- Anaphylactoid reactions (1%)
- Cough [1]
- Headache
- Hyperesthesia [1]
- Myalgia
- Tremor (1–6%) [5]
- Xerostomia (1%) [1]

FOSINOPRIL

Trade name: Monopril (Bristol-Myers Squibb)
Other common trade names: *Acenor-M; Dynacil; Fosinorm; Fozitec; Staril; Vasopril*
Indications: Hypertension
Category: Angiotensin-converting enzyme (ACE) inhibitor; Antihypertensive
Half-life: 11.5 hours
Clinically important, potentially hazardous interactions with: amiloride, spironolactone, triamterene

Reactions

Skin
- Angioedema (<1%) [2]
- Bullous pemphigoid
- Dermatitis [1]
- Diaphoresis (<1%)
- Edema (<1%)
- Eosinophilic fasciitis [1]
- Eosinophilic vasculitis
- Exfoliative dermatitis
- Flu-like syndrome (<1%)
- Flushing
- Pemphigus [1]
- Pemphigus foliaceus [1]
- Photosensitivity (<1%)
- Pruritus (<1%) [1]
- Rash (sic) (<1%) [1]
- Scleroderma [1]
- Urticaria (<1%)
- Vasculitis

Other
- Ageusia (<1%)
- Anaphylactoid reactions
- Cough [2]
- Dysgeusia (<1%) [1]
- Gynecomastia
- Headache
- Myalgia (<1%)
- Paresthesias (<1%)
- Tinnitus
- Tremor (<1%)
- Xerostomia (<1%)

FUROSEMIDE*

Trade name: Lasix (Sanofi-Aventis)
Other common trade names: *Apo-Furosemide; Discoid; Dryptal; Edenol; Frusid; Furorese; Furoside; Fusid; Henexal; Lasilix; Novo-Semide; Urex; Uritol*
Indications: Edema
Category: Antihypertensive; Sulfonamide loop diuretic
Half-life: 0.5–1 hour
Clinically important, potentially hazardous interactions with: amikacin, amyl nitrite, digoxin, gentamicin, kanamycin, neomycin, streptomycin, tobramycin

Reactions

Skin
- Acute febrile neutrophilic dermatosis (Sweet's syndrome) [1]
- Acute generalized exanthematous pustulosis (AGEP) [1]
- Bullous eruption (<1%) [17]
- Bullous pemphigoid [11]
- Diaphoresis
- Epidermolysis bullosa [2]
- Erythema multiforme (<1%) [3]
- Erythema nodosum [1]
- Exanthems (0.2–12%) [8]
- Exfoliative dermatitis [3]
- Flushing [1]
- Grinspan's syndrome** [1]
- Lichenoid eruption [2]
- Linear IgA dermatosis [2]
- Lupus erythematosus [1]
- Photosensitivity (1–10%) [2]
- Phototoxicity [3]
- Porokeratosis (disseminated superficial) [1]
- Pruritus (<1%) [3]
- Purpura [3]
- Pustules [3]
- Rash (sic) (<1%)
- Side effects (sic) [2]
- Stevens–Johnson syndrome [2]
- Toxic epidermal necrolysis [2]
- Urticaria [3]
- Vasculitis [7]

Eyes
- Dyschromatopsia
- Periorbital edema [1]

Other
- Acute intermittent porphyria
- Anaphylactoid reactions [2]
- Headache
- Injection-site erythema (<1%)
- Injection-site pain
- Paresthesias
- Porphyria [1]
- Porphyria cutanea tarda [3]
- Pseudolymphoma [1]
- Pseudoporphyria cutanea tarda [1]
- Thrombophlebitis
- Tinnitus
- Ulcerative stomatitis [1]
- Xerostomia [1]

***Note:** Furosemide is a sulfonamide and can be absorbed systemically. Sulfonamides can produce severe, possibly fatal, reactions such as toxic epidermal necrolysis and Stevens–Johnson syndrome

****Note:** Grinspan's syndrome is the triad of oral lichen planus, diabetes mellitus, and hypertension

GEMFIBROZIL

Trade name: Lopid (Pfizer)
Other common trade names: *Bolutol; Decrelip; Fibrocit; Gemlipid; Gen-Fibro; Gevilon Uno; Jezil; Lipur; Nu-Gemfibrozil*
Indications: Hyperlipidemia
Category: Antihyperlipidemic
Half-life: 1.5 hours
Clinically important, potentially hazardous interactions with: atorvastatin, bexarotene, cyclosporine, dicumarol, ezetimibe, fluvastatin, lovastatin, pravastatin, rosuvastatin, simvastatin, warfarin

Reactions

Skin
- Abscess
- Acanthosis nigricans
- Angioedema
- Basal cell carcinoma
- Dermatitis (0.4%) [1]
- Dermatomyositis (<1%)
- Eczema (1.9%)
- Erythema multiforme
- Exanthems (3%) [2]
- Exfoliative dermatitis (<1%)
- Ichthyosis
- Lichen planus
- Lupus erythematosus
- Melanoma
- Petechiae
- Pruritus (0.8%) [1]
- Psoriasis [2]
- Rash (sic) (1.7%)
- Raynaud's phenomenon (<1%) [1]
- Seborrhea
- Thickening
- Urticaria (0.1%) [1]
- Vasculitis (<1%) [1]
- Xerosis

Hair
- Hair – alopecia
- Hair – hirsutism

Nails
- Nails – discoloration [1]
- Nails – growth

Other
- Anaphylactoid reactions
- Death [2]
- Dysgeusia (<1%)
- Headache
- Hyperesthesia (<1%)
- Myalgia (<1%) [2]
- Myositis
- Paresthesias (<1%)
- Polymyositis [1]
- Pseudolymphoma [1]
- Rhabdomyolysis [20]

GLIMEPIRIDE*

Trade name: Amaryl (Sanofi-Aventis)
Indications: Non-insulin dependent diabetes type II
Category: Second generation sulfonylurea antidiabetic
Half-life: 5–9 hours

Reactions

Skin
- Allergic reactions (sic) (<1%)
- Diaphoresis
- Edema (<1%)
- Erythema (<1%)
- Exanthems (<1%)
- Exfoliative dermatitis
- Lichenoid eruption [1]
- Photosensitivity (<1%)
- Pruritus (<1%)
- Psoriasis [1]
- Rash (sic) (<1%) [1]
- Urticaria (<1%)

Other
- Headache
- Porphyria cutanea tarda

***Note:** Glimepiride is a sulfonamide and can be absorbed systemically. Sulfonamides can produce severe, possibly fatal, reactions such as toxic epidermal necrolysis and Stevens–Johnson syndrome

GLIPIZIDE*

Trade names: Glucotrol (Pfizer); Metaglip (Bristol-Myers Squibb)
Other common trade names: *Glibenese; Glipid; Glyde; Melizide; Mindiab; Minidiab; Minodiab*
Indications: Non-insulin dependent diabetes type II
Category: Second generation sulfonylurea antidiabetic
Half-life: 2–4 hours

Reactions

Skin
- Eczema
- Edema (<1%)
- Erythema (<1%)
- Exanthems (<1%)
- Exfoliative dermatitis
- Flushing (<1%)
- Grinspan's syndrome** [1]
- Lichenoid eruption
- Photosensitivity (1–10%)
- Phototoxicity [1]
- Pigmented purpuric eruption [1]
- Pruritus (<3%)
- Psoriasis (induced) [1]
- Purpura
- Rash (sic) (1–10%)
- Urticaria (1–10%)

Other
- Headache
- Hyperesthesia (<3%)
- Myalgia (<3%)
- Oral lichen planus [1]
- Paresthesias (<3%)
- Porphyria (coproporphyria-like) [1]
- Porphyria cutanea tarda

***Note:** Glipizide is a sulfonamide and can be absorbed systemically. Sulfonamides can produce severe, possibly fatal, reactions such as toxic epidermal necrolysis and Stevens–Johnson syndrome

****Note:** Grinspan's syndrome: the triad of oral lichen planus, diabetes mellitus, and hypertension

GLYBURIDE

Synonyms: glibenclamide; glybenclamide
Trade names: Diabeta (Sanofi-Aventis); Glucovance (Bristol-Myers Squibb); Glynase (Pfizer); Micronase (Pfizer)
Other common trade names: *Albert (Glyburide); Daonil; Euglucan; Euglucon; Glimel; Glucal; Hemi-Daonil; Med-Glibe; Miglucan; Norboral*
Indications: Non-insulin dependent diabetes type II
Category: Second generation sulfonylurea antidiabetic
Half-life: 5–16 hours
Clinically important, potentially hazardous interactions with: bosentan

Glucovance is glyburide and metformin

Reactions

Skin
- Allergic reactions (sic) (0.21%) [1]
- Angioedema
- Bullous eruption [1]
- Eczema
- Erythema (1–5%) [1]
- Exanthems (1–5%) [3]
- Exfoliative dermatitis
- Flushing [2]
- Lichenoid eruption
- Linear IgA dermatosis [2]
- Pemphigus [1]
- Peripheral edema [1]
- Photosensitivity (1–10%) [7]
- Pruritus (1–10%) [3]
- Psoriasis [2]
- Purpura [2]
- Rash (sic) (1–10%)
- Urticaria (1–5%) [5]
- Vasculitis [5]
- Vesiculobullous eruption [1]

Eyes
- Eyelid edema [1]

Other
- Dysgeusia
- Headache
- Hypersensitivity (generalized) [1]
- Myalgia
- Paresthesias (<1%)
- Porphyria cutanea tarda

***Note:** Glyburide is a sulfonamide and can be absorbed systemically. Sulfonamides can produce severe, possibly fatal, reactions such as toxic epidermal necrolysis and Stevens–Johnson syndrome

GOLDENSEAL

Scientific name: *Hydrastis canadensis*
Family: Ranunculaceae
Trade and other common names: Eye balm; Goldenroot; Ground raspberry; Huanglian; Indian dye; Jaundice root; Orange root; Warnera; Yellow puccoon; Yellow root
Category: Antiarrhythmic; Antihistamine; Antimicrobial; Vasodilator
Purported indications and other uses: Oral: Anorexia, fever, hemorrhoids, hemorrhage, liver disorders, menstrual disorders, rhinitis, upper respiratory tract infections, urinary tract infections. **Topical:** Acne, conjunctivitis, dandruff, earache, eczema, eye inflammation, herpes, itching, mouthwash, rash, ringworm, tinnitus, wounds
Half-life: N/A

Reactions

Skin
- Photosensitivity [1]
- Phototoxicity [1]

Other
- Death (overdose)
- Depression (overdose)
- Hallucinations (overdose)
- Mucosal irritation
- Seizures (overdose)

GUANABENZ

Other common trade names: *Rexitene; Wytens*
Category: Alpha-2-adrenoceptor blocker; Antihypertensive
Half-life: 7–10 hours

Reactions

Skin
- Edema (<3%)
- Hyperhidrosis
- Pruritus (<3%)
- Rash (sic) (<3%)

Other
- Dysgeusia (<3%)
- Gynecomastia (<3%)
- Headache
- Sialorrhea
- Xerostomia (28%) [1]

GUANADREL

Indications: Hypertension
Category: Adrenergic agonist; Antihypertensive
Half-life: 5–45 hours (terminal)

Reactions

Skin
- Peripheral edema (28.6%)

Other
- Dizziness [1]
- Fatigue [1]
- Glossitis (8.4%)
- Headache
- Paresthesias (25.1%)
- Xerostomia (1.7%)

GUANETHIDINE

Trade name: Ismelin (Novartis)
Other common trade names: *Apo-Guanethidine; Ismeline*
Indications: Hypertension
Category: Alpha-2-adrenoceptor blocker; Antihypertensive
Half-life: 5–10 days
Clinically important, potentially hazardous interactions with: amitriptyline, amoxapine, benzphetamine, chlorpromazine, clomipramine, desipramine, doxepin, **ephedra**, ephedrine, imipramine, insulin, insulin glargine, minoxidil, nortriptyline, protriptyline, trimipramine

Reactions

Skin
- Dermatitis
- Exanthems
- Fixed eruption [1]
- Lupus erythematosus
- Peripheral edema (>10%)
- Purpura
- Urticaria
- Vasculitis [1]

Hair
- Hair – alopecia

Other
- Dizziness [1]
- Glossitis (5%)
- Headache
- Myalgia
- Paresthesias (16%)
- Priapism
- Sialorrhea
- Xerostomia (1–10%)

GUANFACINE

Trade name: Tenex (ESP)
Other common trade names: *Entulic; Estulic*
Indications: Hypertension
Category: Alpha-2-adrenoceptor blocker; Antihypertensive
Half-life: 10–30 hours

Reactions

Skin
Dermatitis (<3%)
Diaphoresis (<3%) [3]
Edema
Exanthems
Exfoliative dermatitis
Peripheral edema [1]
Pruritus (<3%) [1]
Purpura (<3%)
Rash (sic) [1]
Urticaria

Hair
Hair – alopecia

Other
Dysgeusia (<3%) [1]
Hallucinations [1]
Headache
Paresthesias (<3%)
Sialorrhea
Tinnitus
Xerostomia (47%) [6]

HAWTHORN (FRUIT, LEAF, FLOWER EXTRACT)

Scientific names: *Crataegus laevigata; Crataegus monogyna; Crataegus oxyacantha; Crataegus pentagyna*
Family: Rosaceae
Trade and other common names: Arterio-K; Aubepine; Basticrat; Born; Cardiplant; Cordapur; Coronal; Cratamed; Harthorne; Haw; HeartCare (Nature's Way); Hedgethorne; Maythorn; Nan Shanzha; Naranocor; Regulacor; Shanzha; Thorn Plum; Whitethorn
Category: Improves cardiac function
Purported indications and other uses: Amenorrhea, arrhythmias, atherosclerosis, diuretic, hyperlipidemia, hypertension, hypotension, sedative, appetite stimulant, arthritis, enteritis, indigestion, sore throats. **TopicalB: boils, sores and ulcers**
Half-life: N/A
Clinically important, potentially hazardous interactions with: digoxin

Note: The American Herbal Products Association (AHPA) gives hawthorn a class 1 safety rating, indicating that it is very safe. However, hawthorn should be used with caution in patients with heart disease

Reactions

Skin

Allergic reactions (sic)
Diaphoresis [1]
Rash (sic) (hands) [2]
Toxicoderma [1]

Other

Dizziness [2]
Hypersensitivity [1]

HEPARIN

Trade name: Hep-Flush (Wyeth)
Other common trade names: *Calcilean; Calciparin; Caprin; Hepalean; Heparin-Leo; Heparine; Liquemin; Uniparin*
Indications: Venous thrombosis, pulmonary embolism
Category: Anticoagulant
Half-life: 1.5 hours
Clinically important, potentially hazardous interactions with: aspirin, bivalirudin, butabarbital, **capsicum**, danaparoid, **dong quai**, **ginger**, **horse chestnut (bark, flower, leaf, seed, red clover**, tirofiban

Reactions

Skin

Allergic reactions (sic) (1–10%) [2]
Angioedema (<1%)
Baboon syndrome [1]
Burning (soles) [1]
Chills
Dermatitis [5]
Erythema
Erythema nodosum
Exanthems [2]
Fixed eruption [1]
Hemorrhage [2]
Lesions (sic) [1]
Livedo reticularis [1]
Necrosis [54]
Peripheral edema [1]
Petechiae [1]
Pruritus (<1%)
Purpura (>10%)
Rash (sic)
Scleroderma [1]
Toxic dermatitis [1]
Toxic epidermal necrolysis [2]
Ulcerations [1]
Urticaria (<1%) [5]
Vasculitis [5]

Hair

Hair – alopecia [2]

Nails

Nails – discoloration

Hematopoietic

Ecchymoses [2]

Other

Anaphylactoid reactions [2]
Gingivitis (>10%)
Headache
Hypersensitivity [13]
Injection-site eczematous eruption (<1%) [4]
Injection-site hematoma
Injection-site induration [4]
Injection-site necrosis (<1%) [4]

Injection-site nodules [1]
Injection-site pain [1]
Injection-site plaques [2]
Injection-site purpura [1]
Injection-site urticaria [1]
Priapism [2]

HYDRALAZINE

Trade names: Apresazide (Novartis); Apresoline (Novartis); Ser-Ap-Es (Novartis)
Other common trade names: *Alphapress; Apdormin; Apresolin; Novo-Hylazin; Nu-Hydral; Solesorin; Stable*
Indications: Hypertension
Category: Antihypertensive; Vasodilator
Half-life: 3–7 hours

Apresazide is hydralazine and hydrochlorothiazide; Ser-Ap-Es is hydralazine, reserpine and hydrochlorothiazide

Reactions

Skin
Acute febrile neutrophilic dermatosis (Sweet's syndrome) [5]
Allergic reactions (sic) [1]
Angioedema (<1%)
Bullous eruption [1]
Chills
Dermatitis (systemic) [1]
Diaphoresis
Edema (<1%)
Erythema nodosum [1]
Exanthems [4]
Fixed eruption (<1%) [1]
Flushing (>10%) [1]
Lupus [2]
Lupus erythematosus (6.7%) [97]
Photosensitivity [1]
Pruritus [1]
Purpura [3]
Pyoderma gangrenosum [1]
Rash (sic) (<1%)
Sjøgren's syndrome [1]
Ulcerations [2]
Urticaria
Vasculitis [9]

Other
Arthralgia [1]
Death
Headache
Hypersensitivity
Myalgia [1]
Oral ulceration [2]
Orogenital ulceration [2]
Paresthesias
Relapsing polychondritis [1]
Tremor

HYDROCHLOROTHIAZIDE

Trade names: Accuretic (Pfizer); Aldactazide (Pfizer); Aldoril (Merck); Atacand HCT (AstraZeneca); Avalide (Bristol-Myers Squibb); Capozide (Par); Diovan (Novartis); Dyazide (GSK); Hyzaar (Merck); Inderide (Wyeth); Lopressor (Novartis); Lotensin (Novartis); Maxzide (Mylan Bertek); Micardis (Boehringer Ingelheim); Microzide (Watson); Moduretic (Merck); Prinzide (Merck); Teveten HCT (Biovail); Uniretic (Schwarz); Vaseretic (Biovail); Zestoretic (AstraZeneca); Ziac (Barr)

Other common trade names: *Apo-Hydro; Clothia; Dichlotride; Diu-Melsin; Diuchlor H; Esidrex; Hydrosaluric; Urozide*

Indications: Edema

Category: Antihypertensive; Thiazide diuretic

Half-life: 5.6–14.8 hours

Clinically important, potentially hazardous interactions with: digoxin, lithium

Aldactazide is spironolactone and hydrochlorothiazide; Aldoril is methyldopa and hydrochlorothiazide; Avalide is irbesartan and hydrochlorothiazide; Capozide is captopril and hydrochlorothiazide; Dyazide is triamterene and hydrochlorothiazide; Maxzide is triamterene and hydrochlorothiazide; Moduretic is amiloride and hydrochlorothiazide; Prinzide is lisinopril and hydrochlorothiazide

Reactions

Skin

- Acute generalized exanthematous pustulosis (AGEP) [1]
- Bullous eruption (<1%)
- Dermatitis [2]
- Diaphoresis [1]
- Erythema annulare centrifugum [2]
- Erythema multiforme (<1%) [1]
- Exanthems [1]
- Exfoliative dermatitis
- Fixed eruption [1]
- Lichenoid eruption [4]
- Lupus erythematosus [14]
- Photosensitivity (<1%) [19]
- Phototoxicity [3]
- Porokeratosis (Mibelli) [1]
- Pruritus (<1%) [2]
- Purpura [6]
- Rash (sic) [1]
- Stevens–Johnson syndrome [1]
- Toxic epidermal necrolysis [2]
- Urticaria [1]
- Vasculitis [2]

Eyes

- Dyschromatopsia

Other

- Depression [1]
- Dysgeusia [1]
- Headache
- Oral lichenoid eruption (erosive) [1]
- Paresthesias
- Pseudoporphyria [1]
- Xerostomia

***Note:** Hydrochlorothiazide is a sulfonamide and can be absorbed systemically. Sulfonamides can produce severe, possibly fatal, reactions such as toxic epidermal necrolysis and Stevens–Johnson syndrome

HYDROFLUMETHIAZIDE*

Other common trade names: *Diademil; Hydravern; Hydrenox; Leodrine; Rivosil; Rontyl*
Indications: Hypertension, edema
Category: Antihypertensive; Thiazide diuretic
Duration of action: 12–24 hours
Clinically important, potentially hazardous interactions with: digoxin, lithium

Reactions

Skin
- Photosensitivity (<1%)
- Purpura
- Rash (sic) (<1%)
- Urticaria
- Vasculitis

Eyes
- Dyschromatopsia

Other
- Dysgeusia
- Paresthesias (<1%)

***Note:** Hydroflumethiazide is a sulfonamide and can be absorbed systemically. Sulfonamides can produce severe, possibly fatal, reactions such as toxic epidermal necrolysis and Stevens–Johnson syndrome

IBUTILIDE

Trade name: Corvert (Pfizer)
Indications: Atrial fibrillation and flutter
Category: Antiarrhythmic class III
Half-life: 2–12 hours

Reactions

Skin
- Bullous eruption
- Dermatitis [1]

Other
- Headache
- Torsades de pointes [1]

INDAPAMIDE*

Trade name: Lozol (Sanofi-Aventis)
Other common trade names: *Dapa-tabs; Fludex; Ipamix; Lozide; Naplin; Natrilix; Pamid*
Indications: Edema
Category: Antihypertensive sulfonamide diuretic
Half-life: 14–18 hours
Clinically important, potentially hazardous interactions with: digoxin, lithium

Reactions

Skin
- Angioedema [3]
- Bullous eruption
- Diaphoresis
- Erythema multiforme [2]
- Exanthems [1]
- Fixed eruption [1]
- Flushing (<5%) [1]
- Necrotizing vasculitis
- Pemphigus foliaceus [1]
- Peripheral edema (<5%)
- Photosensitivity (<1%)
- Pigmentation [1]
- Pruritus (<5%) [2]
- Purpura
- Rash (sic) (<5%) [4]
- Stevens–Johnson syndrome [1]
- Toxic epidermal necrolysis [3]
- Urticaria (<5%) [1]
- Vasculitis (<5%)

Eyes
- Dyschromatopsia

Other
- Anaphylactoid reactions
- Headache
- Paresthesias (<5%)
- Xerostomia (<5%) [2]

***Note:** Indapamide is a sulfonamide and can be absorbed systemically. Sulfonamides can produce severe, possibly fatal, reactions such as toxic epidermal necrolysis and Stevens–Johnson syndrome

IRBESARTAN

Trade names: Avalide (Bristol-Myers Squibb); Avapro (Bristol-Myers Squibb) (Sanofi-Aventis)
Indications: Hypertension
Category: Angiotensin II receptor antagonist; Antihypertensive
Half-life: 11–15 hours

Avalide is irbesartan and hydrochlorothiazide (a sulfonamide)*

Reactions

Skin
- Angioedema [1]
- Chills (<1%)
- Dermatitis (<1%)
- Eczema [1]
- Edema (1–10%)
- Erythema (<1%)
- Facial edema (<1%)
- Flushing (<1%)
- Pemphigus herpetiformis [1]
- Pruritus (<1%)
- Rash (sic) (1–10%)
- Urticaria (<1%)

Eyes
- Eyelid edema [1]

Hematopoietic
- Ecchymoses (<1%)

Other
- Cough [2]
- Headache
- Oral lesions (<1%)
- Paresthesias (<1%)
- Tremor (<1%)

***Note:** Avalide contains a sulfonamide which can be absorbed systemically. Sulfonamides can produce severe, possibly fatal, reactions such as toxic epidermal necrolysis and Stevens–Johnson syndrome

ISOETHARINE

Trade names: Arm-a-Med; Beta-2; Bronkomed; Dey-Lute
Other common trade names: *Asthmalitan; Numotac*
Indications: Bronchial asthma
Category: Adrenergic agonist; Bronchodilator; Sympathomimetic
Half-life: N/A

Reactions

Other
Anaphylactoid reactions [1]
Trembling (1–10%)
Tremor
Xerostomia (1–10%)

ISOPROTERENOL

Trade names: Aerolone; Isuprel (Hospira)
Other common trade names: *Isopro; Isuprel Mistometer; Isuprel Nebulimetro; Saventrine; Vapo-Iso*
Indications: Bronchospasm, ventricular arrhythmias
Category: Adrenergic bronchodilator; Sympathomimetic
Half-life: 2.5–5 minutes

Reactions

Skin
Diaphoresis (1–10%)
Edema
Flushing (1–10%)
Pruritus
Rash (sic)
Urticaria

Other
Headache
Oral lesions [1]
Salivary changes (sic) (pinkish-red) (>10%)
Trembling
Tremor
Xerostomia (>10%)

ISOSORBIDE DINITRATE

Synonyms: ISD; ISDN
Trade names: Dilatrate-SR (Schwarz); Isordil (Wyeth); Sorbitrate (AstraZeneca)
Other common trade names: *Apo-ISDN; Cedocard; Coradur*
Indications: Angina pectoris
Category: Antianginal; Vasodilator
Half-life: 4 hours (oral)
Clinically important, potentially hazardous interactions with: sildenafil

Reactions

Skin
- Diaphoresis
- Edema (<1%) [1]
- Exanthems [1]
- Flushing (>10%) [1]
- Pallor
- Peripheral edema [1]

Other
- Headache
- Xerostomia

ISOSORBIDE MONONITRATE

Synonym: ISMN
Trade names: Imdur (Schering); Ismo; Monoket (Schwarz)
Indications: Angina pectoris
Half-life: ~4 hours
Clinically important, potentially hazardous interactions with: sildenafil

Reactions

Skin
- Diaphoresis
- Edema (<1%)
- Flushing (>10%) [1]
- Peripheral edema [1]
- Pruritus (<1%)
- Rash (sic) (<1%)

Other
- Headache
- Hyperesthesia (<1%)
- Tooth disorder (sic) (<1%)

ISOXSUPRINE

Trade names: Vasodilan; Voxsuprine
Other common trade names: *Duvadilan; Isoxine; Sincen; Vasolan; Vasosuprina; Xuprin*
Indications: Peripheral vascular disease, Raynaud's phenomenon
Category: Peripheral vasodilator
Half-life: N/A

Reactions

Skin
- Dermatitis [1]

ISRADIPINE

Trade name: DynaCirc (Reliant)
Other common trade names: *Dynacirc SRO; Lomir; Lomir SRO; Prescal; Vascal*
Indications: Hypertension
Category: Antihypertensive; Calcium channel blocker
Half-life: 8 hours
Clinically important, potentially hazardous interactions with: epirubicin, imatinib, phenytoin

Reactions

Skin
- Diaphoresis (<1%)
- Edema (7.2%) [6]
- Exanthems (1.5%) [2]
- Flushing (2–9%) [8]
- Peripheral edema
- Pruritus (<6%) [1]
- Rash (sic) (1.5%)
- Urticaria (<1%)

Other
- Dizziness (9%) [1]
- Gingival hypertrophy (<1%)
- Headache (9%) [1]
- Oral lesions (6%) [1]
- Paresthesias (<1%)
- Torsades de pointes [1]
- Xerostomia (<1%)

LABETALOL

Trade names: Normozide; Trandate (Prometheus)
Other common trade names: *Abetol; Amipress; Hybloc; Ipolab; Labrocol; Presolol; Salmagne*
Indications: Hypertension
Category: Antihypertensive; Beta-adrenoceptor blocker
Half-life: 3–8 hours

Normozide is labetalol and hydrochlorothiazide

Note: Cutaneous side effects of beta-receptor blockaders are clinically polymorphous. They apparently appear after several months of continuous therapy. Atypical psoriasiform, lichen planus-like, and eczematous chronic rashes are mainly observed. (1983): Hödl St, *Z Hautkr* (German) 1:58, 17

Reactions

Skin
- Angioedema [1]
- Dermatitis [1]
- Diaphoresis (<1%)
- Eczema
- Edema (<2%)
- Exanthems (1–5%) [4]
- Exfoliative dermatitis
- Facial edema
- Flushing (19%) [1]
- Lichen planus (bullous) [1]
- Lichenoid eruption [5]
- Lupus erythematosus [3]
- Peripheral edema
- Pigmentation (slate-gray) [1]
- Pityriasis rubra pilaris [2]

Pruritus (1–10%) [3]
Psoriasis (exacerbation) [3]
Purpura [1]
Rash (sic) (<1%)
Raynaud's phenomenon (<1%)
Side effects (sic) (5.5%) [2]
Urticaria [1]
Xerosis

Hair

Hair – alopecia (reversible) [1]

Other

Anaphylactoid reactions [2]
Dysgeusia (1–10%) [1]
Headache
Hyperesthesia (1%)
Hypersensitivity
Myalgia [4]
Paresthesias (7%) [2]
Peyronie's disease [1]
Priapism
Scalp tingling [3]
Xerostomia

LEVOBETAXOLOL

Trade name: Betaxon (Alcon)
Other common trade name: *L-betaxolol*
Indications: Chronic open-angle glaucoma, ocular hypertension
Category: Antiglaucoma ; Beta-adrenoceptor blocker (ophthalmic)
Half-life: 20 hours

Reactions

Skin

Dermatitis (<2%)
Infections (<2%)
Psoriasis (<2%)
Rash (sic)
Xerosis

Hair

Hair – alopecia (<2%)

Eyes

Ocular transient discomfort (11%)

Other

Breast abscess (<2%)
Dysgeusia (<2%)
Tendinitis (<2%)
Tinnitus (<2%)

LEVOBUNOLOL

Trade name: Betagan (Allergan)
Other common trade names: *Bunolgan; Gotensin; Vistagan; Vistagen*
Indications: Glaucoma, ocular hypertension
Category: Beta-adrenoceptor blocker (ophthalmic)
Half-life: N/A

Reactions

Skin

Dermatitis [7]
Erythema
Lichen planus [1]

Pruritus (<1%)
Rash (sic) (<1%)
Urticaria

Hair

Hair – alopecia (1–10%)

Eyes

Ocular burning [1]
Ocular stinging [1]

Other

Headache
Hypersensitivity

***Note:** Peak effect: 1–7 days

LIDOCAINE

Synonym: lignocaine
Trade names: Anamantle HC (Doak); Anestacon; ELA-Max (Ferndale); EMLA (AstraZeneca); Lidoderm (Endo); Xylocaine (AstraZeneca)
Other common trade names: *Dentipatch; DermaFlex; Dilocaine; Lidodan; Lidoject-2; Octocaine; Xylocard*
Indications: Ventricular arrhythmias, topical anesthesia
Category: Anesthetic; Antiarrhythmic
Half-life: terminal: 1.5–2 hours
Clinically important, potentially hazardous interactions with: amprenavir, cimetidine, fosamprenavir

Reactions

Skin

Allergic reactions (sic) [1]
Angioedema [3]
Bullous eruption
Dermatitis [25]
Eczema [3]
Edema (<1%) [1]
Erythema [1]
Erythema multiforme [1]
Exanthems [2]
Exfoliative dermatitis [2]
Fixed eruption [2]
Lupus erythematosus [1]
Pigmentation [1]
Pruritus (<1%) [2]
Purpura
Rash (sic) (<1%)
Shivering (1–10%)
Stevens–Johnson syndrome [1]
Urticaria [3]

Other

Acute intermittent porphyria
Anaphylactoid reactions [5]
Application-site edema [1]
Application-site erythema [2]
Application-site pallor [1]
Death [2]
Embolia cutis medicamentosa (Nicolau syndrome) [1]
Headache
Hypersensitivity [6]
Injection-site pain
Injection-site phlebitis
Paresthesias (<1%) [1]
Seizures [4]
Stomatitis [1]
Tinnitus
Tremor

LISINOPRIL

Trade names: Prinivil (Merck); Prinzide (Merck); Zestoretic (AstraZeneca); Zestril (AstraZeneca)
Other common trade names: *Acerbon; Alapril; Apo-Lisinopril; Carace; Coric; Prinil; Tensopril; Vivatec*
Indications: Hypertension
Category: Angiotensin-converting enzyme (ACE) inhibitor; Antihypertensive
Half-life: 12 hours
Clinically important, potentially hazardous interactions with: amiloride, **garlic**, spironolactone, triamterene

Prinzide is lisinopril and hydrochlorothiazide; Zestoretic is lisinopril and hydrochlorothiazide

Reactions

Skin

Angioedema (<1%) [19]
Bullous eruption [1]
Diaphoresis (<1%)
Edema (1%)
Erythema (1%)
Exanthems (3%) [4]
Facial edema (<1%)
Flushing (<1%) [3]
Kaposi's sarcoma [1]
Lichenoid eruption [1]
Lupus erythematosus
Pemphigus
Pemphigus foliaceus [2]
Peripheral edema (<1%) [1]
Photosensitivity (<1%)
Pruritus (1.2%) [1]
Purpura [2]
Rash (sic) (1.5%) [5]
Rosacea [1]
Stevens–Johnson syndrome
Telangiectasia [1]
Toxic epidermal necrolysis
Ulcerations (ischemic skin ulcer) [1]
Urticaria (<1%) [2]
Vasculitis (<1%) [1]

Hair

Hair – alopecia (<1%)

Other

Anaphylactoid reactions (<1%)
Cough [3]
Dysesthesia (<1%)
Dysgeusia [1]
Headache
Mastodynia (<1%)
Myalgia (0.5%)
Paresthesias (0.8%)
Tinnitus
Tremor
Xerostomia (<1%)

LOSARTAN

Synonyms: DuP 753; MK 594
Trade names: Cozaar (Merck); Hyzaar (Merck)
Indications: Hypertension
Category: Angiotensin II receptor antagonist; Antihypertensive
Half-life: 2 hours

Hyzaar is losartan and hydrochlorothiazide

Reactions

Skin
- Angioedema (<1%) [9]
- Dermatitis (<1%)
- Diaphoresis (<1%)
- Edema (<1%)
- Erythema (<1%)
- Exanthems
- Facial edema (<1%)
- Flushing (<1%) [1]
- Photosensitivity (<1%)
- Pruritus (<1%)
- Purpura [2]
- Rash (sic) (<1%)
- Urticaria (<1%)
- Xerosis (<1%)

Hair
- Hair – alopecia (<1%)

Hematopoietic
- Ecchymoses (<1%)

Other
- Ageusia [2]
- Anaphylactoid reactions (<1%)
- Aphthous stomatitis [1]
- Dysgeusia (<1%) [1]
- Fetal death [1]
- Headache
- Hyperesthesia (<1%)
- Myalgia (1%)
- Oral ulceration [1]
- Paresthesias (<1%) [1]
- Pseudolymphoma [2]
- Tremor (<1%)
- Xerostomia (<1%)

LOVASTATIN

Trade names: Advicor (Kos); Altocor; Mevacor (Merck)
Other common trade names: *Apo-Lovastatin; Lovalip; Mevinacor; Mevinolin; Nergadan; Rovacor; Taucor*
Indications: Hypercholesterolemia
Category: Antihyperlipidemic; HMG-CoA reductase inhibitor
Half-life: 1–2 hours
Clinically important, potentially hazardous interactions with: atazanavir, azithromycin, bosentan, cholestyramine, clarithromycin, cyclosporine, delavirdine, erythromycin, fenofibrate, fosamprenavir, gemfibrozil, **grapefruit Juice**, imatinib, itraconazole, itraconazole, tacrolimus, telithromycin, verapamil

Reactions

Skin
- Erythema
- Erythema multiforme
- Exanthems (<5%) [3]
- Flushing [1]
- Lupus erythematosus [3]
- Pruritus (5.2%) [2]
- Purpura [1]
- Rash (sic) (5.2%) [3]
- Stevens–Johnson syndrome [1]
- Toxic epidermal necrolysis
- Urticaria
- Vasculitis

Hair
- Hair – alopecia (>1%)

Other
- Dysgeusia (0.8%)

Gynecomastia (1–10%) [1]
Headache [1]
Hypersensitivity
Hyposmia [1]
Myalgia (1–10%) [3]
Paresthesias (>1%)
Pseudolymphoma [1]
Rhabdomyolysis [19]
Stomatitis
Xerostomia (>1%)

MECAMYLAMINE

Trade name: Inversine (Targacept)
Other common trade name: *Mevasine*
Indications: Hypertension
Category: Antihypertensive; Peripherally acting antiadrenergic ganglion blocker
Half-life: N/A

Reactions

Skin

Angioedema

Other

Abdominal pain
Depression
Dizziness
Glossitis
Paresthesias
Seizures
Trembling
Tremor
Xerostomia

MECLOFENAMATE

Trade name: Meclofenamate
Other common trade names: *Kyroxan; Melvon; Movens*
Indications: Arthritis
Category: Nonsteroidal anti-inflammatory (NSAID)
Half-life: 2 hours
Clinically important, potentially hazardous interactions with: methotrexate

Reactions

Skin

Angioedema (<1%) [1]
Bullous eruption
Edema (>1%)
Erythema multiforme (<1%) [3]
Erythema nodosum (<1%)
Erythroderma [1]
Exanthems (1–9%) [4]
Exfoliative dermatitis (<1%) [2]
Fixed eruption (<1%) [3]
Hot flashes (<1%)
Lupus erythematosus
Peripheral edema
Photosensitivity [2]
Pruritus (1–10%) [3]
Psoriasis (exacerbation) [1]
Purpura (>1%) [4]
Rash (sic) (3–9%) [1]
Stevens–Johnson syndrome (<1%)
Toxic epidermal necrolysis (<1%)

Urticaria (>1%) [2]
Vasculitis [3]
Vesiculobullous eruption [2]

Hair

Hair – alopecia (<1%)

Other

Aphthous stomatitis [1]
Dysgeusia (<1%)
Headache
Hypersensitivity [1]
Oral ulceration
Paresthesias (<1%)
Porphyria
Serum sickness
Stomatitis (1–3%)
Tinnitus
Xerostomia

METHAZOLAMIDE

Trade name: Methazolamide
Indications: Glaucoma
Category: Carbonic anhydrase inhibitor; Sulfonamide diuretic
Half-life: ~14 hours

Reactions

Skin

Exanthems (<1%) [2]
Photosensitivity
Pruritus
Purpura
Rash (sic)
Stevens–Johnson syndrome [3]
Toxic epidermal necrolysis
Urticaria [1]
Vasculitis

Other

Anosmia (<1%)
Dysgeusia (>10%) (metallic taste)
Hypersensitivity (<1%)
Paresthesias (<1%)
Tinnitus
Trembling
Xerostomia (<1%)

METHYCLOTHIAZIDE

Other common trade names: *Enduron-M; Thiazidil; Urimor*
Indications: Hypertension
Category: Antihypertensive; Thiazide diuretic
Half-life: N/A
Clinically important, potentially hazardous interactions with: digoxin, lithium

Reactions

Skin

Erythema multiforme
Exanthems
Photosensitivity (<1%)
Purpura
Rash (sic) (<1%)
Stevens–Johnson syndrome
Urticaria

Other
Anaphylactoid reactions
Dysgeusia
Paresthesias (<1%)

***Note:** Methyclothiazide is a sulfonamide and can be absorbed systemically. Sulfonamides can produce severe, possibly fatal, reactions such as toxic epidermal necrolysis and Stevens–Johnson syndrome

METHYLDOPA

Trade names: Aldoclor (Merck); Aldomet; Aldoril
Other common trade names: *Amodopa; Densul; Dopamet; Equibar; Hydopa; Medimet; Nu-Medopa; Polinal; Presinol; Prodopa*
Indications: Hypertension
Category: Alpha-adrenoceptor blocker; Antihypertensive
Half-life: 1.7 hours
Clinically important, potentially hazardous interactions with: ephedrine

Aldoril is methyldopa and hydrochlorothiazide

Reactions

Skin
Cheilitis [1]
Eczema [3]
Edema
Erythema multiforme (<1%) [2]
Erythema nodosum [1]
Exanthems (3%) [3]
Fixed eruption [1]
Granulomas [1]
Lichen planus [3]
Lichenoid eruption [9]
Lupus erythematosus (<1%) [13]
Papulovesicular eruption [1]
Peripheral edema [1]
Petechiae [1]
Photosensitivity [2]
Pigmentation [3]
Pruritus [1]
Purpura [1]
Rash (sic) (<1%)
Seborrheic dermatitis [3]
Stevens–Johnson syndrome [1]
Toxic epidermal necrolysis
Urticaria [2]
Vasculitis [1]

Hair
Hair – alopecia

Other
Acute intermittent porphyria
Black tongue (<1%) [1]
Galactorrhea [1]
Glossodynia
Gynecomastia (<1%)
Headache
Hypersensitivity [1]
Myalgia
Oral lichenoid eruption [3]
Oral mucosal eruption [1]
Oral ulceration [5]
Paresthesias (<1%)
Parkinsonism
Xerostomia (1–10%) [1]

METIPRANOLOL

Trade names: Disorat; Metipranolol; OptiPranolol (Bausch & Lomb); Ripix; Turoptin
Indications: Open angle glaucoma, ocular hypertension
Category: Beta-adrenergic blocker; ophthalmic
Half-life: N/A
Clinically important, potentially hazardous interactions with: reserpine

Reactions

Skin
- Allergic reactions (sic)
- Dermatitis [1]
- Psoriasis [1]
- Rash (sic)

Eyes
- Blepharitis
- Conjunctivitis
- Eye pain
- Eyelid burning
- Eyelid dermatitis
- Eyelid edema
- Eyelid stinging
- Ocular burning [1]
- Ocular stinging [1]
- Tearing
- Uveitis [12]

Other
- Anxiety
- Arthralgia
- Asthenia
- Cough
- Depression
- Dizziness
- Headache
- Myalgia

METOLAZONE*

Trade name: Zaroxolyn (Celltech)
Other common trade names: *Barolyn; Diondel; Metenix 5; Normelan; Xuret*
Indications: Hypertension, edema
Category: Antihypertensive; Sulfonamide diuretic
Half-life: 6–20 hours
Clinically important, potentially hazardous interactions with: digoxin, lithium

Reactions

Skin
- Chills (1–10%)
- Edema (<2%)
- Exanthems
- Exfoliative dermatitis
- Photosensitivity (<2%)
- Pruritus (<2%)
- Purpura (<1%)
- Rash (sic) (<2%)
- Stevens–Johnson syndrome
- Toxic epidermal necrolysis [1]
- Urticaria (<2%)
- Vasculitis [2]
- Xerosis (<2%)

Eyes
- Dyschromatopsia (<2%)

Other

Anaphylactoid reactions (<2%)
Dysgeusia (<2%)
Headache
Paresthesias (<2%)
Tinnitus
Xerostomia (<2%)

***Note:** Metolazone is a sulfonamide and can be absorbed systemically. Sulfonamides can produce severe, possibly fatal, reactions such as toxic epidermal necrolysis and Stevens–Johnson syndrome

METOPROLOL

Trade names: Lopressor (Novartis); Toprol XL (AstraZeneca)
Other common trade names: *Beloc-Zoc; Betaloc; Betazok; Kenaprol; Mycol; Prolaken; Ritmolol; Seloken-Zok; Selozok*
Indications: Hypertension, angina pectoris
Category: Antihypertensive; Beta-adrenoceptor blocker
Half-life: 3–4 hours
Clinically important, potentially hazardous interactions with: clonidine, epinephrine, verapamil

Lopressor HCT is metoprolol and hydrochlorothiazide

Note: Cutaneous side effects of beta-receptor blockaders are clinically polymorphous. They apparently appear after several months of continuous therapy. Atypical psoriasiform, lichen planus-like, and eczematous chronic rashes are mainly observed. (1983): Hödl St, *Z Hautkr* (German) 58, 17

Reactions

Skin

Angioedema [1]
Diaphoresis
Eczema [2]
Edema
Erythema multiforme
Exanthems (1%) [1]
Exfoliative dermatitis
Hyperkeratosis (palms and soles)
Lichenoid eruption [3]
Lupus erythematosus [1]
Peripheral edema (1%)
Pigmentation
Pityriasis rubra pilaris [1]
Prurigo [1]
Pruritus (1–5%) [2]
Psoriasis (induction and aggravation of) [10]
Purpura
Rash (sic) (<5%)
Raynaud's phenomenon (<1%) [2]
Scleroderma [1]
Toxic epidermal necrolysis
Urticaria
Xerosis

Hair

Hair – alopecia [1]

Nails

Nails – dystrophy
Nails – onycholysis
Nails – pigmentation
Nails – transverse depression [1]

Eyes

Oculo-mucocutaneous syndrome [1]

Other
- Dysgeusia
- Gangrene (feet) [1]
- Headache
- Oral lichenoid eruption
- Paresthesias
- Peyronie's disease [5]
- Polymyositis [1]
- Scalp tingling [1]
- Tinnitus

MEXILETINE

Trade name: Mexitil (Boehringer Ingelheim)
Other common trade names: *Mexihexal; Mexilen; Mexitec*
Indications: Ventricular arrhythmias
Category: Antiarrhythmic class I B
Half-life: 10–12 hours
Clinically important, potentially hazardous interactions with: caffeine

Reactions

Skin
- Acute generalized exanthematous pustulosis (AGEP) [1]
- Diaphoresis (<1%)
- Edema (3.8%)
- Exanthems [8]
- Exfoliative dermatitis (<1%)
- Facial edema [1]
- Hot flashes (<1%)
- Lupus erythematosus (<1%)
- Pruritus [1]
- Purpura
- Rash (sic) (3.8%)
- Stevens–Johnson syndrome (<1%)
- Urticaria [2]
- Xerosis (<1%)

Hair
- Hair – alopecia (<1%)

Other
- Dysgeusia (<1%) [1]
- Headache
- Paresthesias (3.8%)
- Pseudolymphoma [1]
- Salivary changes (<1%)
- Tinnitus
- Trembling (1–10%)
- Tremor (12.6%)
- Xerostomia (2.8%)

MIDODRINE

Trade name: Proamatine (Shire)
Other common trade names: *Amatine; Gutron; Metligine; Midon*
Indications: Orthostatic hypotension, urinary incontinence
Category: Alpha agonist; Antihypotensive; Vasopressor
Half-life: ~3–4 hours

Reactions

Skin
- Chills (5%)
- Erythema multiforme
- Flushing (1–10%)
- Pruritus (13%) [2]
- Rash (sic) (2.4%)
- Xerosis (2%)

Hair
- Hair – pili torti [2]

Other
- Aphthous stomatitis
- Headache
- Hyperesthesia
- Pain (5%)
- Paresthesias (13–18%) [3]
- Xerostomia (1–10%)

MINOXIDIL

Trade names: Loniten (Par); Rogaine (topical) (Pfizer)
Other common trade names: *Alopexy; Apo-Gain; Hairgaine; Lonolox; Lonoten; Minoximen; Regaine*
Indications: Hypertension, androgenetic alopecia
Category: Antihypertensive; Vasodilator
Half-life: 4.2 hours
Clinically important, potentially hazardous interactions with: guanethidine

Note: For topical reaction patterns, I have added a bracket [T]

Reactions

Skin
- Acne [1]
- Allergic reactions (sic) [T]
- Bullous eruption (<1%) [2]
- Dermatitis (7.4%) [T] [12]
- Eczema [2]
- Edema (>10%) [T] [1]
- Erythema [T]
- Erythema multiforme [1]
- Erythroderma [1]
- Exanthems [4]
- Flushing [T]
- Folliculitis [T] [1]
- Lupus erythematosus [2]
- Peripheral edema (7%)
- Pigmentation
- Pruritus [T] [3]
- Pyogenic granuloma [1]
- Rash (sic) (<1%)
- Seborrhea [T]
- Stevens–Johnson syndrome (<1%) [1]
- Sunburn (<1%)
- Urticaria
- Xerosis

Hair
- Hair – alopecia [T] [2]
- Hair – hirsutism (in women) (100%) [2]
- Hair – hypertrichosis (80–100%) [20]
- Hair – pigmentation [2]

Other
- Anaphylactoid reactions [1]
- Anosmia [1]
- Dysgeusia [T] [1]

Gynecomastia
Headache
Mastodynia (<1%)
Paresthesias
Polymyositis [1]
Tendinitis [T]

MIRTAZAPINE

Trade name: Remeron (Organon)
Indications: Depression
Category: Alpha-2-adrenoceptor blocker; Tetracyclic antidepressant
Half-life: 20–40 hours
Clinically important, potentially hazardous interactions with: telithromycin

Reactions

Skin
Acne
Allergic reactions (sic) [1]
Cellulitis
Chills
Diaphoresis [1]
Edema (1–10%) [1]
Exfoliative dermatitis
Facial edema
Flu-like syndrome (1–10%) [1]
Herpes simplex
Peripheral edema (1–10%) [1]
Petechiae
Photosensitivity
Pruritus
Rash (sic) (1–10%) [1]
Seborrhea
Ulcerations
Xerosis

Other
Ageusia
Anxiety [1]
Aphthous stomatitis
Arthralgia [2]
Dysgeusia
Fatigue [2]
Glossitis (1–10%)
Gynecomastia
Headache [1]
Hyperesthesia
Mastodynia
Myalgia (1–10%) [1]
Oral candidiasis
Paresthesias [1]
Parosmia
Phlebitis
Restless legs syndrome [3]
Rhabdomyolysis [1]
Serotonin syndrome [4]
Sialorrhea
Stomatitis
Tendon rupture
Tongue edema
Tongue pigmentation
Tremor (1–10%) [1]
Vaginitis
Xerostomia (25%) [1]

MOEXIPRIL

Trade names: Uniretic (Schwarz); Univasc (Schwarz)
Indications: Hypertension
Category: Angiotensin-converting enzyme (ACE) inhibitor; Antihypertensive
Half-life: 1 hour
Clinically important, potentially hazardous interactions with: amiloride, spironolactone, triamterene

Uniretic is moexipril and hydrochlorothiazide

Reactions

Skin
- Adverse effects (sic) [1]
- Angioedema (<1%) [1]
- Diaphoresis (<1%)
- Exanthems (1.6%)
- Flushing (1.6%) [1]
- Pemphigus (<1%)
- Pemphigus foliaceus [1]
- Peripheral edema (1–10%) [1]
- Photosensitivity (<1%)
- Pruritus (1–10%)
- Rash (sic) (1.6%)
- Urticaria (<1%)

Hair
- Hair – alopecia (1–10%)

Other
- Anaphylactoid reactions (<1%)
- Cough [2]
- Dysgeusia (<1%)
- Headache
- Myalgia (1.3%)
- Xerostomia (<1%)

MORICIZINE

Trade name: Ethmozine (Shire)
Indications: Ventricular arrhythmias
Category: Antiarrhythmic class I
Half-life: 3–4 hours

Reactions

Skin
- Diaphoresis (2–5%)
- Exanthems (<1%)
- Pruritus (<2%)
- Rash (sic) (<1%)
- Urticaria (<2%)
- Xerosis (<2%)

Eyes
- Periorbital edema (1–10%)

Other
- Dysgeusia (<2%)
- Hyperesthesia (2–5%)
- Oral lesions [1]
- Paresthesias (2–5%)
- Thrombophlebitis (<2%)
- Tinnitus
- Tongue edema (<2%)
- Xerostomia (2–5%) [2]

NADOLOL

Trade names: Corigard; Corzide (Monarch)
Other common trade names: *Apo-Nadolol; Farmagard; Nadic; Solgol; Syn-Nadolol*
Indications: Hypertension, angina pectoris
Category: Antianginal; Antihypertensive; Beta-adrenoceptor blocker
Half-life: 10–24 hours
Clinically important, potentially hazardous interactions with: clonidine, epinephrine, verapamil

Corzide is nadolol and bendroflumethiazide*

Note: Cutaneous side effects of beta-receptor blockaders are clinically polymorphous. They apparently appear after several months of continuous therapy. Atypical psoriasiform, lichen planus-like, and eczematous chronic rashes are mainly observed. (1983): Hödl St, *Z Hautkr* (German) 58, 17

Reactions

Skin
- Bullous pemphigoid [1]
- Diaphoresis (<1%) [1]
- Eczema
- Edema (1–5%)
- Erythema multiforme
- Exanthems (<1%) [1]
- Exfoliative dermatitis
- Facial edema (<1%)
- Hyperkeratosis (palms and soles)
- Infiltrative dermatitis of the scalp [1]
- Lichenoid eruption [1]
- Lupus erythematosus
- Pityriasis rubra pilaris [1]
- Pruritus (1–5%)
- Psoriasis [4]
- Pustules [1]
- Rash (sic) (1–5%)
- Raynaud's phenomenon (2%) [2]
- Toxic epidermal necrolysis
- Urticaria
- Xerosis

Hair
- Hair – alopecia [1]

Nails
- Nails – dystrophy
- Nails – onycholysis
- Nails – pigmentation

Eyes
- Oculo-mucocutaneous syndrome [1]

Other
- Dysgeusia
- Gingivitis [1]
- Headache
- Numbness (fingers and toes) (>5%)
- Oral lichenoid eruption
- Oral mucosal eruption (<1%) [1]
- Paresthesias (>5%)
- Peyronie's disease [1]
- Tinnitus
- Xerostomia (<1%) [1]

***Note:** Bendroflumethiazide is a sulfonamide and can be absorbed systemically. Sulfonamides can produce severe, possibly fatal, reactions such as toxic epidermal necrolysis and Stevens–Johnson syndrome

NEBIVOLOL

Trade name: Nebilet (Menarini)
Indications: Hypertension
Category: Beta-adrenoceptor blocker
Half-life: 8 hours

Reactions

Other
Myalgia
Paresthesias [1]

NESIRITIDE

Trade name: Natrecor (Scios)
Indications: Acutely decompensated congestive heart failure
Category: Human B-type natriuretic peptide; Vasodilator
Half-life: 18 minutes

Reactions

Skin
Diaphoresis (>1%)
Pruritus (>1%)
Rash (sic) (>1%)

Other
Back pain
Cough (>1%)
Headache
Leg cramps (>1%)
Paresthesias (>1%)
Phlebitis
Tremor (>1%)

NIACIN

Synonym: nicotinic acid
Trade names: Advicor (Kos); Niacor (Upsher-Smith); Niaspan (Merck); Nicobid; Nicotinex; Slo-Niacin (Upsher-Smith)
Other common trade names: *Apo-Nicotinamide; I*; IV; Nia-Bid; Niac; Niacels; Nicobion; Nicotinex; Nicovital; Pepeom Amide; Vitamin B_3*
Indications: Hyperlipidemia
Category: Antihyperlipidemic
Half-life: 45 minutes
Clinically important, potentially hazardous interactions with: atorvastatin, selenium, selenium

Reactions

Skin
- Acanthosis nigricans (8%) [17]
- Dermatitis [1]
- Erythema [1]
- Exanthems (<3%) [3]
- Fixed eruption (<1%) [1]
- Flushing (1–30%) [22]
- Ichthyosis [1]
- Keratoses [1]
- Pigmentation [1]
- Pruritus (1–5%) [10]
- Rash (sic) (<1%) [4]
- Scaling [1]
- Urticaria [1]
- Xerosis

Other
- Anaphylactoid reactions
- Burning mouth syndrome [1]
- Fatigue [1]
- Gingivitis [1]
- Headache [1]
- Myalgia [4]
- Paresthesias (1–10%) [2]
- Toothache [1]
- Xerostomia

NICARDIPINE

Trade name: Cardene (Roche)
Other common trade names: *Antagonil; Dagan; Loxen; Nicardal; Nicodel; Ranvil; Ridene; Rydene*
Indications: Angina, hypertension
Category: Antianginal; Antimigraine; Calcium channel blocker
Half-life: 2–4 hours
Clinically important, potentially hazardous interactions with: epirubicin, imatinib, telithromycin

Reactions

Skin
- Allergic reactions (sic)
- Edema (1%)
- Exanthems
- Flushing (5.6%) [2]
- Peripheral edema (7.1%) [2]
- Rash (sic) (1.2%) [3]
- Side effects (sic) [1]
- Urticaria [3]

Other
- Erythromelalgia [2]
- Gingival hypertrophy (<1%)
- Headache
- Myalgia (1%) [1]
- Paresthesias (1%)
- Parotitis
- Tinnitus
- Xerostomia (1.4%)

NIFEDIPINE

Trade names: Adalat (Bayer); Procardia (Pfizer)
Other common trade names: *Adalate; Apo-Nifed; Aprical; Calcilat; Coracten; Corogal; Corotrend; Nifecor; Nu-Nifed; Pidilat*
Indications: Angina, hypertension
Category: Antianginal; Antimigraine; Calcium channel blocker
Half-life: 2–5 hours
Clinically important, potentially hazardous interactions with: epirubicin, imatinib, rifampin, ritonavir

Reactions

Skin
- Acute generalized exanthematous pustulosis (AGEP) [2]
- Angioedema (<1%) [2]
- Bullous eruption [2]
- Chills (2%)
- Dermatitis (<2%)
- Diaphoresis (<2%) [2]
- Edema [2]
- Erysipelas [2]
- Erythema [2]
- Erythema multiforme [4]
- Erythema nodosum [2]
- Exanthems (1%) [9]
- Exfoliative dermatitis (<1%) [5]
- Facial edema (1%)
- Fixed eruption [3]
- Flushing (3–25%) [5]
- Lichenoid eruption [3]
- Lupus erythematosus [3]
- Pemphigoid nodularis [1]
- Pemphigus foliaceus [1]
- Peripheral edema [8]
- Photosensitivity [6]
- Prurigo nodularis [1]
- Pruritus (<2%) [3]
- Purpura (<2%) [3]
- Rash (sic) (<3%) [2]
- Shaking (2%)
- Side effects (sic) [1]
- Stevens–Johnson syndrome [3]
- Telangiectasia [3]
- Toxic epidermal necrolysis [2]
- Ulcerations [1]
- Urticaria (<1%) [7]
- Vasculitis [3]

Hair
- Hair – alopecia (1%) [4]
- Hair – pigmentation [1]

Nails
- Nails – dystrophy [1]

Eyes
- Periorbital edema (1%) [1]

Other
- Dysgeusia (<1%)
- Erythromelalgia (<0.5%) [4]
- Gingival hypertrophy (6–10%) [38]
- Gynecomastia (<1%) [3]
- Headache
- Myalgia (<1%)
- Paresthesias (<3%) [1]
- Parosmia
- Parotitis
- Tinnitus
- Tremor (2–8%)
- Xerostomia (<3%)

NIMODIPINE

Trade name: Nimotop (Bayer)
Other common trade names: *Admon; Periplum; Vasotop*
Indications: Subarachnoid hemorrhage
Category: Calcium channel blocker
Half-life: 3 hours
Clinically important, potentially hazardous interactions with: epirubicin, imatinib

Reactions

Skin
- Acne (<1%)
- Acute generalized exanthematous pustulosis (AGEP) [1]
- Diaphoresis (<1%)
- Edema (2%)
- Exanthems (2.4%) [1]
- Flushing (2.1%)
- Peripheral edema
- Pruritus (<1%)
- Purpura
- Rash (sic) (3%)

Hair
- Hair – alopecia [1]

Other
- Headache

NISOLDIPINE

Trade name: Sular (First Horizon)
Other common trade names: *Baymycard; Syscor*
Indications: Hypertension
Category: Antihypertensive; Calcium channel blocker
Half-life: 7–12 hours
Clinically important, potentially hazardous interactions with: epirubicin, imatinib

Reactions

Skin
- Acne (<1%)
- Angioedema
- Cellulitis (<1%)
- Chills (<1%)
- Diaphoresis (<1%)
- Exanthems (<1%) [1]
- Exfoliative dermatitis (<1%)
- Facial edema (<1%)
- Flu-like syndrome (<1%)
- Flushing [1]
- Herpes simplex (<1%)
- Herpes zoster (<1%)
- Peripheral edema (22%) [1]
- Petechiae (<1%)
- Photosensitivity
- Pigmentation (<1%)
- Pruritus (<1%)
- Pustules (<1%)
- Rash (sic) (2%)
- Side effects (sic) [1]
- Ulcerations (<1%)
- Urticaria (<1%)
- Xerosis (<1%)

Hair
- Hair – alopecia (<1%)

Hematopoietic
Ecchymoses (<1%)

Other
Dysgeusia (<1%)
Gingival hypertrophy (<1%)
Glossitis (<1%)
Gynecomastia (<1%)
Headache
Hyperesthesia (<1%)
Hypersensitivity
Oral ulceration (<1%)
Paresthesias (<1%)
Tremor (<1%)
Vaginitis (<1%)
Xerostomia (<1%)

NITROGLYCERIN

Synonyms: glyceryl trinitrate; nitroglycerol; NTG

Trade names:
- Buccal tablets
- Lingual aerosol: Nitrolingual (First Horizon)
- Oral capsules: Nitrocap; Nitrocine; Nitroglyn; Nitrospan
- Oral tablets: Klavikordal; Niong; Nitronet; Nitrong
- Parenteral: Nitro-Bid; Nitroject; Nitrol; Nitrostat (Pfizer); Tridil
- Sublingual tablets: Nitrostat (Pfizer)
- Topical ointment: Nitrol; Nitrong; Nitrostat (Pfizer)
- Topical transdermal systems: Deponit; Minitran (3M); Nitrocine; Nitrodisc; Nitrodur; Transderm-Nitro (Various pharmaceutical companies.)

Other common trade names: *Cardinit; Corditrine; Lenitral; Nitradisc; Nitroglin; Suscard; Sustac*
Indications: Acute angina
Category: Antianginal; Antihypertensive; Vasodilator
Half-life: 1–4 minutes
Clinically important, potentially hazardous interactions with: acetylcysteine, alteplase, sildenafil

Reactions

Skin
Allergic reactions (sic) (<1%)
Angioedema [1]
Cyanosis
Dermatitis (to topical systems) (<1%) [23]
Diaphoresis (<1%)
Eczema [2]
Edema
Erythema (to transdermal delivery system) [1]
Erythema multiforme [1]
Erythroderma [1]
Exanthems
Exfoliative dermatitis (1–10%) [1]
Flushing (>10%) [1]
Pallor
Peripheral edema (<1%)
Purpura [2]
Rash (sic) (1–10%)
Rosacea (exacerbation) [1]
Urticaria

Other
Anaphylactoid reactions (from perianal application) [1]
Headache (42%) [1]
Oral burn (from sublingual)
Xerostomia (<1%)

OCTREOTIDE

Trade name: Sandostatin (Novartis)
Other common trade names: *Sandostatina; Sandostatine*
Indications: Diarrhea
Category: Antihypoglycemic; Antihypotensive; Growth hormone suppressant; Somatostatin analog
Half-life: 1.5 hours

Reactions

Skin
Allergic reactions (sic)
Cellulitis (1–4%)
Diaphoresis
Edema (1–10%)
Exanthems [1]
Flushing (1–4%) [1]
Granulomas [1]
Petechiae (1–4%)
Pruritus (1–4%)
Purpura (1–4%)
Rash (sic) (<1%)
Raynaud's phenomenon (1–4%)
Urticaria (1–4%)

Hair
Hair – alopecia (<1%) [2]

Other
Anaphylactoid reactions
Galactorrhea (1–4%)
Gynecomastia (1–4%)
Headache
Hyperesthesia (<1%)
Injection-site erythema (1%)
Injection-site granuloma [1]
Injection-site pain (7.5%)
Injection-site reactions (sic)
Thrombophlebitis (1–4%)
Vaginitis (1–4%)
Xerostomia

OLMESARTAN

Trade name: Benicar (Sankyo)
Indications: Hypertension
Category: Angiotensin II receptor antagonist
Half-life: ~13 hours
Clinically important, potentially hazardous interactions with: ephedra, garlic, ginseng, lithium

Reactions

Skin
Angioedema
Facial edema
Flu-like syndrome (>1%)

Peripheral edema (>0.5)
Rash (sic) (0.5%)
Upper respiratory infection (>1%)

Other
Arthralgia (>0.5%)
Back pain (>1%)
Bone or joint pain (>0.5%)
Cough (0.7%)
Dizziness (3%) [2]
Myalgia (>0.5%)
Pain (>0.5%)

PAPAVERINE

Trade names: Genabid; Pavabid; Pavatine
Other common trade names: *Angioverin; Optenyl; Pameion; Papaverine 60; Papaverini; Pavagen; Pavased*
Indications: Peripheral and cerebral ischemia
Category: Peripheral vasodilator
Half-life: 0.5–2 hours

Reactions

Skin
Diaphoresis (<1%)
Exanthems
Fixed eruption [1]
Flushing (<1%)
Pruritus (<1%)
Pyogenic granuloma [1]
Rash (sic)
Toxic epidermal necrolysis [1]
Urticaria

Other
Headache
Injection-site thrombophlebitis (<1%)
Priapism (11%) [3]
Xerostomia (<1%)

PENBUTOLOL

Trade name: Levatol (Schwarz)
Other common trade names: *Betapresin; Betapressin*
Indications: Hypertension
Category: Antihypertensive; Beta-adrenoceptor blocker
Half-life: 5 hours
Clinically important, potentially hazardous interactions with: clonidine, epinephrine, verapamil

Note: Cutaneous side effects of beta-receptor blockaders are clinically polymorphous. They apparently appear after several months of continuous therapy. Atypical psoriasiform, lichen planus-like, and eczematous chronic rashes are mainly observed. (1983): Hödl St, *Z Hautkr* (German) 1:58, 17

Reactions

Skin
- Allergic reactions (sic) (1–5%) [1]
- Diaphoresis (1.6%)
- Exanthems (1–5%) [1]
- Flushing (1–5%) [1]
- Peripheral edema
- Pruritus
- Psoriasis
- Purpura
- Rash (sic)

Hair
- Hair – alopecia

Nails
- Nails – pigmentation

Other
- Dysgeusia
- Headache
- Paresthesias
- Peyronie's disease

PENTOXIFYLLINE

Trade names: Pentoxil (Upsher-Smith); Trental (Sanofi-Aventis)
Other common trade names: *Apo-Pentoxifylline; Artal; Azupentat; Elorgan; Hemovas; Pentoxi; Pexal; Torental*
Indications: Peripheral vascular disease, intermittent claudication
Category: Blood viscosity reducing agent
Half-life: 0.4–0.8 hours

Reactions

Skin
- Allergic reactions (sic) [1]
- Angioedema (<1%) [1]
- Diaphoresis
- Edema (<1%)
- Exanthems
- Flushing (2%) [2]
- Pruritus (<1%) [1]
- Purpura
- Rash (sic) (<1%)
- Urticaria

Nails
- Nails – brittle (<1%)

Other
- Anxiety [1]
- Dysgeusia (<1%)
- Dysphagia [2]
- Headache
- Paresthesias [1]
- Serum sickness [1]
- Sialorrhea (<1%)
- Tremor
- Xerostomia (<1%) [1]

PERINDOPRIL

Trade name: Aceon (Solvay)
Other common trade names: *Acertil; Coversum; Coversyl; Prexum*
Indications: Hypertension
Category: Angiotensin-converting enzyme (ACE) inhibitor; Antihypertensive
Half-life: 1.5–3 hours

Reactions

Skin
- Allergic reactions (sic) (1.3%) [1]
- Angioedema (<1%) [2]
- Chills (<1%)
- Diaphoresis (0.3–1%)
- Edema (3.9%)
- Erythema (0.3–1%)
- Exanthems
- Facial edema (<1%)
- Herpes simplex (0.3–1%)
- Palmar–plantar pustulosis [1]
- Pemphigus foliaceus [1]
- Pruritus (1–10%)
- Psoriasis (<1%)
- Purpura (<0.1%)
- Rash (sic) (1–10%) [1]
- Xerosis (0.3–1%)

Hematopoietic
- Ecchymoses (0.3–1%)

Other
- Anaphylactoid reactions (<1%) [1]
- Cough [3]
- Dysgeusia (<1%)
- Headache
- Myalgia (<1%)
- Paresthesias (2.3%)
- Vaginitis (0.3–1%)
- Xerostomia (0.3–1%)

PHENOXYBENZAMINE

Trade name: Dibenzyline (Wellspring)
Other common trade names: *Dibenyline; Dibenzyran*
Indications: Pheochromocytoma
Category: Alpha-adrenoceptor blocker; Antihypertensive
Half-life: 24 hours
Clinically important, potentially hazardous interactions with: epinephrine

Reactions

Skin
- Allergic reactions (sic) [1]
- Dermatitis [1]

Other
- Priapism [1]
- Xerostomia (1–10%)

PHENTOLAMINE

Trade name: Regitine (Novartis)
Other common trade names: *Regitin; Rogitene; Rogitine*
Indications: Hypertensive episodes in pheochromocytoma
Category: Alpha-adrenoceptor blocker; Antihypertensive; Diagnostic aid (pheochromocytoma)
Half-life: 19 minutes

Reactions

Skin
Flushing (1–10%)

Other
Priapism

PHENYLEPHRINE

Trade names: Dura-Vent; Neo-Synephrine; Prolex-D; Rynatan (MedPointe); Tussi-12D (MedPointe)
Other common trade names: *Dionephrine; Novahistine; Prefrin Liquifilm*
Indications: Nasal congestion, glaucoma, hypotension
Category: Alpha-adrenoceptor blocker; Mydriatic ophthalmic agent
Half-life: 2.5 hours
Clinically important, potentially hazardous interactions with: epinephrine, furazolidone, phenelzine, tranylcypromine

Reactions

Skin
Dermatitis [15]
Erythroderma [1]
Pallor
Stinging (from nasal or ophthalmic preparations) (1–10%)

Eyes
Blepharoconjunctivitis [4]
Conjunctivitis [1]
Ocular allergic reactions (sic) [1]
Periorbital dermatitis [3]
Periorbital edema [1]

Other
Headache
Hypersensitivity [1]
Injection-site reactions (sic)
Paresthesias
Tremor

PHENYLPROPANOLAMINE

Synonym: PPA
Trade names: Acutrim; BC Cold Powder; Control; Dex-a-Diet; Dexatrim; Diet Gum; Genex; Maigret-50; Phenoxine; Phenyldrine; Prolamine; Propagest; Propandrine; Rhindecon; Spray-U-Thin; St. Joseph Aspirin-Free Cold Tablets (McNeil); Stay Trim; Unitrol; Westrim
Indications: Nasal decongestion, anorexiant
Category: Adrenergic agonist; Anorexiant; Nasal decongestant; Sympathomimetic
Half-life: 3–4 hours
Clinically important, potentially hazardous interactions with: caffeine, ephedra, ephedrine, fluoxetine, fluvoxamine, furazolidone, **guarana**, paroxetine, sertraline, tranylcypromine

Reactions

Skin
Fixed eruption [1]
Pallor

Other
Death [2]
Depression
Rhabdomyolysis [4]
Tremor
Xerostomia

PHENYTOIN

Synonyms: diphenylhydantoin; DPH; phenytoin sodium
Trade names: Dilantin (Pfizer); Phenytek (Mylan Bertek)
Other common trade names: *Di-Hydran; Diphenylan; Epanutin; Fenytoin; Phenhydan; Pyoredol; Zentropil*
Indications: Grand mal seizures
Category: Antiarrhythmic; Hydantoin anticonvulsant
Half-life: 7–42 hours (dose dependent)
Clinically important, potentially hazardous interactions with: amprenavir, aprepitant, chloramphenicol, cimetidine, clorazepate, cyclosporine, delavirdine, diazoxide, disulfiram, dopamine, fluconazole, fluoxetine, fosamprenavir, **ginkgo biloba**, imatinib, indinavir, **influenza Vaccines**, isoniazid, isradipine, itraconazole, meperidine, midazolam, nelfinavir, nelfinavir, ritonavir, saquinavir, solifenacin, **st john's wort**, sucralfate, telithromycin, ticlopidine, vigabatrin

An excellent overview of cutaneous reactions to phenytoin can be found in (1988): Silverman AK+, *J Am Acad Dermatol* 18, 721

Note: About 19% of patients receiving phenytoin develop skin reactions (1983): Rapp RP+, *Neurosurg* 13, 272. They typically develop 10 to 14 days following the start of treatment

Reactions

Skin
Acne [7]
Acute generalized exanthematous pustulosis (AGEP) [2]

Angioedema [2]
Anticonvulsant hypersensitivity syndrome [2]
Bullous eruption [1]
Dermatomyositis [1]
Eosinophilic fasciitis [1]
Epidermolysis bullosa [1]
Erythema multiforme [11]
Erythroderma [4]
Exanthems (6–71%) [15]
Exfoliative dermatitis [12]
Fixed eruption [3]
Heel pad thickening [1]
Lichen planus [1]
Lichenoid eruption [1]
Linear IgA dermatosis [5]
Lupus erythematosus [16]
Lymphoma (<1%) [5]
Mucocutaneous lymph node syndrome (Kawasaki syndrome) [1]
Mycosis fungoides [4]
Necrosis [1]
Pemphigus [1]
Peripheral edema [1]
Pigmentation [1]
Pruritus [6]
Pseudoacanthosis nigricans [1]
Purple glove syndrome [5]
Purpura [4]
Pustules [3]
Rash (sic) (1–10%) [3]
Reticular hyperplasia [2]
Rhinophyma [1]
Scleroderma [1]
Sezary syndrome [1]
Sjøgren's syndrome [1]
Stevens–Johnson syndrome (14%) [27]
Toxic dermatitis [1]
Toxic epidermal necrolysis (2%) [39]
Urticaria [4]
Vasculitis (2%) [6]
Warts [1]

Hair

Hair – alopecia [3]
Hair – hirsutism [5]
Hair – hypertrichosis [2]

Nails

Nails – changes (sic) [2]
Nails – hypoplasia [3]
Nails – onychopathy [1]
Nails – pigmentation [1]

Other

Acromegaloid features [1]
Acute intermittent porphyria [1]
Ageusia [2]
Application-site pain [1]
Coarse facies [2]
Death
Digital malformations [3]
Dyskinesia [2]
Fetal hydantoin syndrome* [7]
Gingival hypertrophy (>10%) [27]
Gynecomastia [1]
Headache
Hypersensitivity** [32]
Injection-site extravasation [1]
Injection-site necrosis [2]
Injection-site pain [1]
Lymphadenopathy [1]
Lymphoproliferative disease [1]
Mucocutaneous eruption [2]
Myalgia [2]
Oral ulceration [1]
Osteomalacia [1]
Paresthesias (<1%) [2]
Periarteritis nodosa [2]
Peyronie's disease
Polyfibromatosis [1]
Polymyositis [1]

Porphyria [1]
Porphyria cutanea tarda [1]
Pseudolymphoma (<1%) [29]
Rhabdomyolysis [2]
Serum sickness [2]
Thrombophlebitis (<1%)

***Note:** The fetal hydantoin syndrome (FHS) – children whose mothers receive phenytoin during pregnancy are born with FHS. The main features of this syndrome are mental and growth retardation, unusual facies, digital and nail hypoplasia, and coarse scalp hair. Occasionally neonatal acne will be present

PINDOLOL

Trade name: Visken (Novartis)
Other common trade names: *Alti-Pindolol; Apo-Pindol; Barbloc; Durapindol; Gen-Pindolol; Nonspi; Pinbetol; Pinden; Syn-Pindol; Vypen*
Indications: Hypertension
Category: Antihypertensive; Beta-adrenoceptor blocker
Half-life: 3–4 hours
Clinically important, potentially hazardous interactions with: clonidine, epinephrine, verapamil

Note: Cutaneous side effects of beta-receptor blockaders are clinically polymorphous. They apparently appear after several months of continuous therapy. Atypical psoriasiform, lichen planus-like, and eczematous chronic rashes are mainly observed. (1983): Hödl St, *Z Hautkr* (German) 1:58, 17

Reactions

Skin
Diaphoresis (2%)
Eczema
Edema (6%)
Erythema multiforme
Exanthems
Exfoliative dermatitis
Hyperkeratosis (palms and soles)
Lichenoid eruption [2]
Lupus erythematosus [1]
Peripheral edema
Pityriasis rubra pilaris [1]
Pruritus (1–5%) [1]
Psoriasis [5]
Purpura
Rash (sic) (1–10%)
Raynaud's phenomenon [2]
Toxic epidermal necrolysis
Urticaria
Xerosis

Hair
Hair – alopecia

Nails
Nails – dystrophy
Nails – onycholysis

Eyes
Oculo-mucocutaneous syndrome [1]

Other
Dysgeusia
Myalgia [1]
Oral lichenoid eruption
Paresthesias (3%)
Peyronie's disease [1]

PIRBUTEROL

Trade name: Maxair (3M)
Other common trade names: *Exirel; Spirolair; Zeisin Autohaler*
Indications: Asthma, bronchospasm
Category: Beta-2-adrenoceptor blocker; Bronchodilator
Half-life: 2–3 hours

Reactions

Skin
- Edema
- Pruritus
- Purpura (< 1%)
- Rash (sic)

Hair
- Hair – alopecia

Other
- Dysgeusia (1–10%)
- Glossitis
- Headache
- Paresthesias (< 1%)
- Trembling (> 10%)
- Xerostomia

POLYTHIAZIDE*

Trade names: Minizide (Pfizer); Renese (Pfizer)
Other common trade names: *Drenusil; Nephril*
Indications: Hypertension, edema
Category: Antihypertensive; Thiazide diuretic
Half-life: N/A
Clinically important, potentially hazardous interactions with: digoxin, lithium

Minizide is prazosin and polythiazide

Reactions

Skin
- Exanthems
- Photosensitivity (< 1%)
- Purpura
- Rash (sic) (< 1%)
- Urticaria
- Vasculitis

Other
- Paresthesias

***Note:** Polythiazide is a sulfonamide and can be absorbed systemically. Sulfonamides can produce severe, possibly fatal, reactions such as toxic epidermal necrolysis and Stevens–Johnson syndrome

PRAVASTATIN

Trade name: Pravachol (Bristol-Myers Squibb)
Other common trade names: *Elisor; Lipostat; Pravasin; Pravasine; Selectin; Selektine; Selipran*
Indications: Hypercholesterolemia
Category: Antihyperlipidemic; HMG-CoA reductase inhibitor
Half-life: ~2–3 hours
Clinically important, potentially hazardous interactions with: azithromycin, clarithromycin, cyclosporine, erythromycin, gemfibrozil, imatinib

Reactions

Skin
- Allergic reactions (sic) [1]
- Angioedema
- Dermatomyositis [1]
- Eczema (generalized) [1]
- Erythema multiforme
- Exanthems
- Flu-like syndrome
- Flushing [1]
- Lichenoid eruption [2]
- Lupus erythematosus
- Neuroleptic malignant syndrome [1]
- Photosensitivity
- Pruritus [2]
- Purpura
- Rash (sic) (1–10%) [7]
- Stevens–Johnson syndrome
- Toxic epidermal necrolysis
- Urticaria
- Vasculitis

Hair
- Hair – alopecia [1]
- Hair – broken-off patches of scalp hair (greenish) [1]

Other
- Anaphylactoid reactions
- Dysgeusia (<1%)
- Gynecomastia [1]
- Headache
- Hypersensitivity
- Myalgia (2.7%) [6]
- Myositis [1]
- Paresthesias
- Polymyositis [1]
- Porphyria cutanea tarda [1]
- Rhabdomyolysis [9]
- Stomatitis

PRAZOSIN

Trade names: Minipress (Pfizer); Minizide (Pfizer)
Other common trade names: *Alti-Prazosin; Apo-Prazo; Duramipress; Eurex; Hypovase; Nu-Prazo; Peripress; Pratisol; Pressin*
Indications: Hypertension
Category: Alpha-adrenoceptor blocker; Antihypertensive
Half-life: 2–4 hours
Clinically important, potentially hazardous interactions with: epinephrine

Minizide is prazosin and polythiazide

Reactions

Skin
- Angioedema [1]
- Diaphoresis (<1%) [2]
- Edema (1–4%) [1]
- Exanthems (1–5%) [1]
- Lichen planus (<1%)
- Lichenoid eruption
- Lupus erythematosus [2]
- Pruritus (<1%) [1]
- Rash (sic) (1–4%) [2]
- Urticaria [1]

Hair
- Hair – alopecia (<1%)

Other
- Anaphylactoid reactions [1]
- Headache
- Myalgia [1]
- Paresthesias (<1%)
- Priapism (<1%) [2]
- Tinnitus
- Xerostomia (1–4%) [3]

PROCAINAMIDE

Trade names: Procan (Pfizer); Procanbid (Pfizer); Pronestyl; Rhythmin
Other common trade names: *Amisalen; Biocoryl; Procan SR; Promine; Ritmocamid*
Indications: Ventricular arrhythmias
Category: Antiarrhythmic class I A
Half-life: 2.5–4.5 hours
Clinically important, potentially hazardous interactions with: abarelix, arsenic, ciprofloxacin, enoxacin, gatifloxacin, lomefloxacin, moxifloxacin, norfloxacin, ofloxacin, sparfloxacin

Reactions

Skin
- Angioedema (<1%) [1]
- Chills (<1%)
- Dermatitis (6%) [1]
- Eczema
- Exanthems (1–8%) [5]
- Flushing (<1%)
- Lichen planus [1]
- Lupus erythematosus (>10%) [169]
- Pruritus (<1%)
- Purpura [3]
- Rash (sic) (<1%)
- Sjøgren's syndrome [1]
- Urticaria (1–5%) [1]
- Vasculitis [4]

Other
- Dysgeusia (3–4%) (bitter taste) [1]
- Myalgia (<1%) [2]
- Oral mucosal eruption (2%) [1]
- Pseudolymphoma [1]
- Torsades de pointes [1]
- Tremor (<1%)

PROPAFENONE

Trade name: Rythmol (Reliant)
Other common trade names: *Arythmol; Norfenon; Normorytmin; Rythmex; Rytmonorm*
Indications: Ventricular arrhythmias
Category: Antiarrhythmic class I C
Half-life: 10–32 hours
Clinically important, potentially hazardous interactions with: digoxin, fosamprenavir, **grapefruit Juice**, ritonavir

Reactions

Skin
- Acne (1%)
- Diaphoresis (1%)
- Edema (<1%)
- Exanthems [1]
- Flushing (<1%)
- Lupus erythematosus (<1%) [2]
- Pruritus (<1%)
- Purpura (<1%)
- Rash (sic) (1–3%)
- Urticaria

Hair
- Hair – alopecia (<1%)

Other
- Death [1]
- Dysgeusia (3–23%) [1]
- Headache
- Injection-site pain (28–90%) [4]
- Oral lesions (>5%) [1]
- Paresthesias (<1%)
- Parosmia (<1%)
- Seizures [1]
- Tinnitus
- Tremor (<1%)
- Xerostomia (2%)

PROPRANOLOL

Trade names: Inderal (Wyeth); Inderide (Wyeth)
Other common trade names: *Acifol; Apsolol; Betabloc; Cinlol; Detensol; Inderalici; Inderex; Novo-Pranol; Prosin; Sinal; Tesnol*
Indications: Hypertension, angina pectoris
Category: Antianginal; Antiarrhythmic class II; Antihypertensive; Beta-adrenoceptor blocker
Half-life: 2–6 hours
Clinically important, potentially hazardous interactions with: cimetidine, clonidine, epinephrine, **eucalyptus**, haloperidol, insulin, insulin glargine, terbutaline, verapamil

Inderide is propranolol and hydrochlorothiazide

Note: Cutaneous side effects of beta-receptor blockaders are clinically polymorphous. They apparently appear after several months of continuous therapy. Atypical psoriasiform, lichen planus-like, and eczematous chronic rashes are mainly observed. (1983): Hödl St, *Z Hautkr* (German) 58, 17

Reactions

Skin
- Acne [1]
- Angioedema [1]
- Bullous eruption [1]
- Cheilitis [1]
- Dermatitis [2]
- Diaphoresis
- Eczema [2]
- Edema
- Erythema (systemic) [1]
- Erythema multiforme [1]
- Exanthems (<1%) [5]
- Exfoliative dermatitis [1]
- Flushing [2]
- Hyperkeratosis (palms and soles)
- Lichenoid eruption [3]
- Lupus erythematosus [2]
- Necrosis
- Pemphigus [2]
- Peripheral edema
- Peripheral skin necrosis [2]
- Photosensitivity [1]
- Phototoxicity [1]
- Pruritus [2]
- Psoriasis [16]
- Purpura [1]
- Pustular psoriasis [2]
- Rash (sic) (1–10%)
- Raynaud's phenomenon (59%) [1]
- Sclerosis [1]
- Stevens–Johnson syndrome [2]
- Toxic epidermal necrolysis [1]
- Toxicoderma [1]
- Urticaria [3]
- Xerosis

Hair
- Hair – alopecia [6]
- Hair – alopecia areata [1]

Nails
- Nails – discoloration [1]
- Nails – onycholysis [1]
- Nails – pitting (psoriasiform) [1]
- Nails – thickening [2]

Other
- Anaphylactoid reactions [1]
- Dupuytren's contracture [1]
- Dysgeusia [1]
- Headache
- Myalgia [1]
- Oral ulceration [1]
- Paresthesias
- Peyronie's disease [6]
- Serum sickness [1]
- Tongue pigmentation [1]
- Xerostomia

PROTAMINE

Indications: Heparin overdose
Category: Heparin antagonist
Duration of action: 2 hours

Reactions

Skin
- Angioedema [1]
- Exanthems [1]
- Flushing (<1%)
- Urticaria [1]

Other
- Anaphylactoid reactions [2]
- Death [1]
- Hypersensitivity (<1%)

PROTAMINE SULFATE

Indications: Heparin overdose
Category: Anticoagulant; Coagulant
Half-life: N/A
Clinically important, potentially hazardous interactions with: None

Reactions

Skin
- Adverse effects (sic) [1]
- Allergic reactions (sic) [12]
- Angioedema [3]
- Erythema [1]
- Flushing
- Rash (sic) [2]
- Urticaria [4]

Other
- Anaphylactoid reactions [35]
- Back pain
- Death [10]
- Headache
- Hypersensitivity [6]
- Malignant hyperthermia [1]
- Rhabdomyolysis [1]

PSEUDOEPHEDRINE

Trade names: Allegra-D (Sanofi-Aventis); Benadryl (Pfizer); Bromfed (Muro); Deconsal; Entex (Andrx); Robitussin-CF (Wyeth); Sudafed (Pfizer); Trinalin (Schering)
Other common trade names: *Balminil; Eltor 120; Maxiphed; Robidrine*
Indications: Nasal congestion
Category: Adrenergic agonist; Nasal decongestant; Sympathomimetic
Half-life: 9–16 hours
Clinically important, potentially hazardous interactions with: bromocriptine, fluoxetine, fluvoxamine, furazolidone, paroxetine, phenelzine, sertraline, tranylcypromine

Reactions

Skin
- Acute generalized exanthematous pustulosis (AGEP) [1]
- Angioedema [2]
- Baboon syndrome [1]
- Dermatitis [3]
- Diaphoresis (1–10%)
- Eczema [1]
- Erythema multiforme [1]
- Erythroderma [1]
- Exanthems [4]
- Exfoliative dermatitis [1]
- Fixed eruption [16]
- Pallor
- Pseudo-scarlatina [1]
- Toxic erythema [1]
- Urticaria [2]

Other
- Headache
- Tinnitus
- Trembling
- Tremor
- Xerostomia

QUINAPRIL

Trade name: Accupril (Pfizer)
Other common trade names: *Accuprin; Accupro; Acuitel; Acupril; Asig; Korec; Quinazil*
Indications: Hypertension
Category: Angiotensin-converting enzyme (ACE) inhibitor; Antihypertensive
Half-life: 1–2 hours
Clinically important, potentially hazardous interactions with: amiloride, spironolactone, triamterene

Reactions

Skin
- Angioedema (<1%) [8]
- Bullous eruption [1]
- Diaphoresis (<1%) [3]
- Edema [2]
- Exanthems [1]
- Exfoliative dermatitis (<1%)
- Facial edema [1]
- Flushing (<1%)
- Pemphigus (<1%)
- Pemphigus foliaceus [1]
- Pemphigus vulgaris [1]
- Peripheral edema [2]
- Photosensitivity (<1%) [1]
- Pruritus (<1%) [7]
- Rash (sic) (1.2%) [5]
- Urticaria (<1%)
- Vasculitis (<1%)

Hair
- Hair – alopecia (<1%)

Other
- Cough [3]
- Dysgeusia [2]
- Headache
- Hypersensitivity
- Myalgia (1.5%)
- Paresthesias (<1%)
- Xerostomia (<1%)

QUINETHAZONE

Trade name: Hydromox
Other common trade name: *Aquamox*
Indications: Hypertension, edema
Category: Sulfonamide diuretic
Half-life: N/A
Clinically important, potentially hazardous interactions with: digoxin, lithium

Reactions

Skin
- Bullous eruption (<1%) [1]
- Exanthems [1]
- Photosensitivity (<1%) [2]
- Pruritus [1]
- Purpura
- Rash (sic) (<1%)
- Urticaria
- Vasculitis

Eyes
- Dyschromatopsia

Other

Hypersensitivity

Paresthesias

Xerostomia

***Note:** Quinethazone is a sulfonamide and can be absorbed systemically. Sulfonamides can produce severe, possibly fatal, reactions such as toxic epidermal necrolysis and Stevens–Johnson syndrome

QUINIDINE

Trade names: Cin-Quin; Quinalan; Quinora
Other common trade names: *Cardine; Gluquine; Kinidin; Quinate; Quini Durules*
Indications: Tachycardia, atrial fibrillation
Category: Antiarrhythmic class I A
Half-life: 6–8 hours
Clinically important, potentially hazardous interactions with: abarelix, amiloride, amiodarone, amprenavir, anisindione, aripiprazole, arsenic, ciprofloxacin, delavirdine, dicumarol, digoxin, duloxetine, enoxacin, fosamprenavir, gatifloxacin, itraconazole, lomefloxacin, moxifloxacin, norfloxacin, ofloxacin, pimozide, pipecuronium, ritonavir, **senna**, sparfloxacin, telithromycin, vecuronium, verapamil, voriconazole, warfarin

Reactions

Skin

Acne [1]
Acute generalized exanthematous pustulosis (AGEP) [2]
Allergic reactions (sic) (1%) [1]
Angioedema (<1%)
Bullous eruption
Dermatitis [3]
Eczema
Erythema multiforme [1]
Exanthems [6]
Exfoliative dermatitis (<1%) [5]
Exudative dermatitis [1]
Fixed eruption [1]
Flushing (<1%) [2]
Granuloma annulare [1]
Lichen planus [7]
Lichenoid eruption [6]
Livedo reticularis (<1%) [5]
Lupus erythematosus (<1%) [34]
Palmar–plantar desquamation [1]
Photosensitivity (<1%) [21]
Pigmentation (<1%) [4]
Pruritus (<1%) [3]
Psoriasis (<1%) [6]
Purpura (1%) [13]
Pustules [1]
Rash (sic) (1–10%)
Side effects (sic) (1%) [1]
Subcorneal pustular dermatosis (Sneddon–Wilkinson) [1]
Toxic epidermal necrolysis [2]
Urticaria (<1%) [1]
Vasculitis (<1%) [4]

Hair

Hair – alopecia [1]

Eyes

Uveitis [1]

Other

Dysgeusia (>10%) (bitter taste)
Headache
Hypersensitivity [1]
Lymphoproliferative disease [1]
Myalgia (<1%)
Oral mucosal eruption [2]

Oral pigmentation [1]
Oral ulceration
Polymyositis [1]
Porphyria [1]
Pseudoporphyria [1]
Sicca syndrome (<1%) [1]
Tinnitus
Torsades de pointes [1]
Tremor (2%)

RAMIPRIL

Trade name: Altace (Monarch)
Other common trade names: *Delix; Hytren; Pramace; Quark; Ramace; Triatec; Tritace; Unipril*
Indications: Hypertension
Category: Angiotensin-converting enzyme (ACE) inhibitor; Antihypertensive
Half-life: 3–17 hours
Clinically important, potentially hazardous interactions with: amiloride, spironolactone, triamterene

Reactions

Skin
Acne [1]
Angioedema (0.3%) [4]
Dermatitis (<1%)
Diaphoresis (<1%) [2]
Dry feeling on face (sic) [1]
Edema (<1%) [1]
Erythema (circumscribed) [1]
Erythema multiforme (<1%)
Exanthems [1]
Flushing [2]
Lichen planus pemphigoides [1]
Pemphigus (<1%) [1]
Pemphigus foliaceus [1]
Photosensitivity (<1%) [3]
Pruritus (<1%) [3]
Purpura (<1%)
Rash (sic) (<1%) [4]
Stevens–Johnson syndrome [1]
Urticaria (<1%)
Vasculitis (<1%) [1]

Hair
Hair – alopecia (1–10%)

Other
Ageusia (<1%)
Anaphylactoid reactions (<1%)
Cough [2]
Dysgeusia (<1%) [1]
Headache
Hypersensitivity (<1%)
Paresthesias (<1%) [1]
Sialorrhea (<1%)
Tinnitus
Tremor (<1%)
Xerostomia (<1%)

RESERPINE

Trade names: Resa; Ser-Ap-Es (Novartis); Serpalan; Serpasil (Novartis); Serpatabs
Other common trade names: *Anserpin; Inerpin; Novo-Reserpine; Reserfia; Sedaraupin; Serpasol; Tionsera*
Indications: Hypertension
Category: Nondiuretic antihypertensive; Rauwolfia alkaloid
Half-life: 50–100 hours
Clinically important, potentially hazardous interactions with: metipranolol

Ser-Ap-Es is reserpine, hydralazine and hydrochlorothiazide

Reactions

Skin
- Bullous eruption [1]
- Edema
- Exanthems
- Flushing
- Lupus erythematosus (exacerbation) [1]
- Peripheral edema (1–10%)
- Pruritus
- Purpura
- Rash (sic) (<1%)
- Toxic epidermal necrolysis [1]
- Urticaria

Other
- Gynecomastia
- Headache
- Parkinsonism
- Sialorrhea
- Xerostomia (>10%)

RETEPLASE

Synonyms: recombinant plasminogen activator; r-PA
Trade name: Retavase (Centocor)
Indications: Acute myocardial infarction
Category: Thrombolytic ; Tissue plasminogen activator
Half-life: 13–16 minutes
Clinically important, potentially hazardous interactions with: abciximab, aspirin, bivalirudin, dipyridamole, piperacillin

Reactions

Skin
- Allergic reactions (sic) (<1%)
- Bleeding
- Purpura

Hematopoietic
- Ecchymoses

Other
- Anaphylactoid reactions (<1%)
- Headache
- Injection-site bleeding (1–10%)

RITODRINE

Trade name: Pre-Par
Indications: Preterm labor
Category: Adrenergic agonist; Tocolytic (uterine relaxant)
Half-life: 1.3–12 hours

Reactions

Skin

- Chills (3–10%)
- Diaphoresis (1–14%) [1]
- Erythema (10–15%)
- Erythema multiforme [1]
- Exanthems
- Pustules (in a pregnant woman with psoriasis) [1]
- Rash (sic) (1–3%) [1]
- Urticaria
- Vasculitis [2]

Other

- Anaphylactoid reactions (1–3%)
- Headache
- Tremor (>10%)

ROSUVASTATIN

Trade name: Crestor (AstraZeneca)
Indications: Hypercholesterolemia, Mixed dyslipidemia
Category: Antihyperlipidemic; HMG-CoA reductase inhibitor
Half-life: ~19 hours
Clinically important, potentially hazardous interactions with: cyclosporine, gemfibrozil, warfarin

Reactions

Skin

- Flu-like syndrome (2.3%)
- Infections
- Peripheral edema (>2%)
- Pruritus (>1%)
- Rash (sic) (>2%)

Hematopoietic

- Ecchymoses (>1%)

Other

- Abdominal pain (>2%)
- Anxiety
- Arthralgia (>2%)
- Asthenia (2.7%)
- Back pain (2.6%)
- Cough (>2%)
- Depression (>2%)
- Dizziness (>2%)
- Headache (6%)
- Myalgia (2.8%)
- Pain (>2%)
- Paresthesias (>2%)
- Rhabdomyolysis
- Rhinitis (2.2%)
- Sinusitis (2%)

SALMETEROL

Trade names: Advair (GSK); Serevent (GSK)
Other common trade names: *Salmeter; Serobid; Zantirel*
Indications: Asthma
Category: Adrenergic agonist; Sympathomimetic bronchodilator
Half-life: 3–4 hours

Reactions

Skin
Angioedema
Eczema [1]
Exanthems
Infections (2–12%) [1]
Pruritus
Rash (sic) (1–3%) [2]
Urticaria (1–3%) [1]

Other
Death [1]
Headache
Hypersensitivity (<1%)
Myalgia (1–3%)
Oral candidiasis [1]
Paresthesias
Trembling
Tremor (1–10) [2]

SIMVASTATIN

Trade name: Zocor (Merck)
Other common trade names: *Denan; Lipex; Liponorm; Lodales; Simovil; Sivastin; Zocord*
Indications: Hypercholesterolemia
Category: Antihyperlipidemic (cholesterol-lowering); HMG-CoA reductase inhibitor
Half-life: 1.9 hours
Clinically important, potentially hazardous interactions with: atazanavir, azithromycin, bosentan, clarithromycin, clarithromycin, cyclosporine, delavirdine, diltiazem, erythromycin, fosamprenavir, gemfibrozil, **grapefruit juice**, imatinib, itraconazole, itraconazole, ritonavir, ritonavir, selenium, selenium, **st john's wort**, tacrolimus, telithromycin, verapamil

Reactions

Skin
Acute generalized exanthematous pustulosis [1]
Angioedema
Cheilitis [1]
Dermatomyositis [2]
Diaphoresis [1]
Eczema [4]
Eosinophilic fasciitis [1]
Erythema multiforme [1]
Erythema nodosum
Exanthems [1]
Flushing [1]
Lichen planus [1]
Lichenoid eruption [1]
Lupus erythematosus [4]
Lupus syndrome [1]
Peripheral edema [1]
Petechiae [1]
Photo-recall [1]
Photosensitivity [5]
Pruritus [2]

Purpura [2]
Pustules
Rash (sic) (1–10%) [3]
Rosacea [1]
Stevens–Johnson syndrome
Toxic epidermal necrolysis
Urticaria
Vasculitis

Hair
Hair – alopecia [5]

Hematopoietic
Thrombocytopenic purpura [1]

Other
Anaphylactoid reactions
Death [2]
Dysgeusia (<1%) [1]
Fatigue (9%) [1]
Gynecomastia
Headache
Hypersensitivity
Myalgia (1–10%) [14]
Myositis [1]
Paresthesias
Polymyositis [1]
Porphyria cutanea tarda [1]
Rhabdomyolysis [28]
Tendinitis [1]

SOTALOL

Trade name: Betapace (Berlex)
Other common trade names: *Beta-Cardone; Betades; Cardol; Sotacor; Sotacor; Sotahexal; Sotalex*
Indications: Ventricular arrhythmias
Category: antiarrhythmic class III; Beta-adrenoceptor blocker
Half-life: 7–18 hours
Clinically important, potentially hazardous interactions with: abarelix, arsenic, ciprofloxacin, enoxacin, gatifloxacin, lomefloxacin, moxifloxacin, norfloxacin, ofloxacin, sparfloxacin

Reactions

Skin
Cold extremities
Diaphoresis (<1%) [1]
Edema (5%)
Exanthems
Irritation (sic)
Lichenoid eruption [1]
Peripheral edema
Photosensitivity (<1%)
Pruritus (1–10%)
Psoriasis [3]
Rash (sic) (3%)
Raynaud's phenomenon (<1%)
Scleroderma [3]
Thickening
Urticaria
Vasculitis [1]

Hair
Hair – alopecia (<1%)

Other
Dysgeusia
Headache
Injection-site extravasation (<1%)
Myalgia [1]
Paresthesias (3%)
Phlebitis (<1%)
Torsades de pointes [1]
Xerostomia (<1%)

SPIRONOLACTONE

Trade names: Aldactazide (Pfizer); Aldactone (Pfizer)
Other common trade names: *Aldopur; Almatol; Diram; Merabis; Novo-Spiroton; Osiren; Spiroctan; Tensin*
Indications: Hyperaldosteronism, hirsutism, hypertension
Category: Diuretic; Potassium-sparing antihypertensive diuretic
Half-life: 78–84 minutes
Clinically important, potentially hazardous interactions with: amiloride, benazepril, captopril, cyclosporine, enalapril, fosinopril, **juniper**, lisinopril, mitotane, moexipril, potassium iodide, quinapril, ramipril, trandolapril, triamterene

Aldactazide is spironolactone and hydrochlorothiazide

Reactions

Skin

Bullous pemphigoid [1]
Chills
Chloasma [1]
Dermatitis [6]
Diaphoresis
Eczema [2]
Erythema
Erythema annulare centrifugum [1]
Erythema multiforme [1]
Exanthems (<5%) [6]
Facial edema [1]
Flushing (<1%)
Graft-versus-host reaction [1]
Lichen planus [1]
Lichenoid eruption [2]
Lupus erythematosus [2]
Melasma [2]
Necrotizing vasculitis
Pemphigus [2]
Photosensitivity
Pigmentation [4]
Pruritus [2]
Purpura
Rash (sic) (1–10%) [2]
Raynaud's phenomenon [1]
Side effects (sic) [1]
Urticaria [2]
Vasculitis [1]
Xerosis (40%) [3]

Hair

Hair – alopecia [2]
Hair – hirsutism

Other

Acute intermittent porphyria
Ageusia
Anaphylactoid reactions
DRESS syndrome [1]
Gynecomastia (<1%) [11]
Headache
Mastodynia [1]
Oral lichen planus [1]
Paresthesias
Xerostomia

STREPTOKINASE

Trade names: Kabikinase (Pfizer); Streptase (AstraZeneca)
Indications: Pulmonary embolism, acute myocardial infarction
Category: Thrombolytic
Half-life: 83 minutes
Clinically important, potentially hazardous interactions with: bivalirudin

Reactions

Skin
- Allergic reactions (sic) (4.4%) [3]
- Angioedema (>10%) [1]
- Bleeding [1]
- Diaphoresis (1–10%)
- Exanthems (1–5%) [2]
- Flushing (<1%)
- Pruritus (1–10%)
- Purpura
- Rash (sic) (1–10%)
- Urticaria (1–5%) [1]
- Vasculitis [7]

Eyes
- Periorbital edema (>10%)

Hematopoietic
- Ecchymoses

Other
- Anaphylactoid reactions (<1%) [1]
- Back pain [1]
- Headache
- Injection-site bleeding [1]
- Injection-site phlebitis
- Serum sickness [5]
- Stomatitis (following local application)
- Tongue edema (with hemorrhagic swelling)

TAMSULOSIN

Trade name: Flomax (Boehringer Ingelheim)
Indications: Benign prostatic hypertrophy
Category: Selective alpha-blocker
Half-life: 9–13 hours
Clinically important, potentially hazardous interactions with: vardenafil

Reactions

Skin
- Angioedema
- Eczema [1]
- Erythema multiforme [1]
- Pruritus
- Rash (sic)

Other
- Dizziness [1]
- Headache
- Priapism [1]
- Rhinitis [1]
- Tooth disorder (sic)

TELMISARTAN

Trade name: Micardis (Boehringer Ingelheim)
Indications: Hypertension
Category: Angiotensin II receptor antagonist; Antihypertensive
Half-life: 24 hours

Reactions

Skin
- Allergic reactions (sic) (<1%)
- Angioedema (>0.3%)
- Dermatitis (>0.3%)
- Diaphoresis (>0.3%)
- Eczema (>0.3%)
- Edema [1]
- Flu-like syndrome (1%)
- Flushing (>0.3%)
- Fungal dermatitis (>0.3%)
- Peripheral edema (1%)
- Pruritus (>0.3%)
- Rash (sic) (>0.3%)

Other
- Cough [1]
- Dizziness [1]
- Headache [1]
- Hyperesthesia (>0.3%)
- Myalgia (1%)
- Paresthesias (>0.3%)
- Xerostomia (>0.3%)

TENECTEPLASE

Trade name: TNKase (Genentech)
Indications: Acute myocardial infarction
Category: Recombinant tissue plasminogen activator; Thrombolytic
Half-life: 90–130 minutes
Clinically important, potentially hazardous interactions with: bivalirudin

Reactions

Skin
- Angioedema (<1%)
- Hematomas (local) (12%)
- Livedo reticularis (<1%)
- Purple glove syndrome (<1%)
- Purpura
- Rash (sic) (<1%)
- Urticaria (<1%)

Hematopoietic
- Ecchymoses

Other
- Anaphylactoid reactions (<1%)
- Gangrene (<1%)
- Rhabdomyolysis (<1%)

TERAZOSIN

Trade name: Hytrin (Abbott)
Other common trade names: *Heitrin; Hitrin; Hytrine; Hytrinex; Itrin; Vicard*
Indications: Hypertension, benign prostatic hypertrophy
Category: Alpha-adrenoceptor blocker; Antihypertensive
Half-life: 12 hours
Clinically important, potentially hazardous interactions with: vardenafil

Reactions

Skin
- Diaphoresis (>1%)
- Edema (1–10%)
- Exanthems [2]
- Facial edema (>1%)
- Flu-like syndrome (<1%)
- Lichenoid eruption [1]
- Peripheral edema (5.5%)
- Phototoxicity [1]
- Pruritus (>1%) [1]
- Rash (sic) (>1%)

Other
- Anaphylactoid reactions
- Headache
- Myalgia (>1%)
- Paresthesias (2.9%)
- Priapism (<1%) [1]
- Tinnitus
- Xerostomia (1–10%)

TERBUTALINE

Trade names: Brethine (aaiPharma); Bricanyl (AstraZeneca)
Other common trade names: *Ataline; Brothine; Bucaril; Butaline; Convon; Respirol; Vacanyl*
Indications: Bronchospasm
Category: Beta-2-adrenergic bronchodilator; Sympathomimetic; Tocolytic
Half-life: 11–16 hours
Clinically important, potentially hazardous interactions with: epinephrine, propranolol

Reactions

Skin
- Dermatitis (irritant) [1]
- Diaphoresis (1–10%)
- Exanthems [1]
- Flushing
- Pruritus [1]
- Urticaria
- Vasculitis [1]

Other
- Dysgeusia (1–10%)
- Headache
- Oral ulceration [1]
- Rhabdomyolysis [1]
- Xerostomia (1–10%)

TICLOPIDINE

Trade name: Ticlid (Roche)
Other common trade names: *Anagregal; Panaldine; Ticlidil; Ticlodix; Ticlodone; Tiklid; Tiklyd*
Indications: To reduce risk of thrombotic stroke
Category: Antithrombotic; Platelet aggregation inhibitor
Half-life: 24 hours
Clinically important, potentially hazardous interactions with: alteplase, **dong quai**, fondaparinux, **garlic**, **ginger**, **ginseng**, **horse chestnut (bark, flower, leaf, seed**, phenytoin, **red clover**

Reactions

Skin
- Acute generalized exanthematous pustulosis (AGEP) [1]
- Angioedema (<1%) [1]
- Bleeding (1–5%) [2]
- Dermatitis [1]
- Diaphoresis (<2%) [1]
- Erythema [1]
- Erythema multiforme (<1%) [1]
- Erythema nodosum (<1%)
- Exanthems (1–11.9%) [6]
- Exfoliative dermatitis (<1%)
- Facial erythema [1]
- Fixed eruption [2]
- Hematomas (2%) [1]
- Lupus [1]
- Lupus erythematosus (positive ANA) (<1%) [1]
- Petechiae (2%) [1]
- Pruritus (1.3%) [3]
- Purpura (2.2%) [2]
- Rash (sic) (5.1%) [2]
- Side effects (sic) (8%) [1]
- Stevens–Johnson syndrome (<1%)
- Toxic erythema [1]
- Urticaria (1–5%) [4]
- Vasculitis (<1%) [1]

Hematopoietic
- Ecchymoses (<1%)
- Thrombocytopenic purpura (1–5%) [23]

Other
- Erythromelalgia [1]
- Fatigue [1]
- Headache
- Serum sickness
- Tinnitus

TIMOLOL

Trade names: Betimol; Blocadren (Merck); CoSopt (Merck); Timoptic (ophthalmic) (Merck)
Other common trade names: *Apo-Timol; Aquanil; Dispatim; Nu-Timolol; Tenopt; Tiloptic; Timacor; Timoptol*
Indications: Hypertension
Category: Antihypertensive; Beta-adrenoceptor blocker
Half-life: 2–2.7 hours
Clinically important, potentially hazardous interactions with: clonidine, epinephrine, verapamil

CoSopt is timolol and dorzolamide; Timolide is timolol and hydrochlorothiazide. Dorzolamide and hydrochlorothiazide are sulfonamides and can be absorbed systemically. Sulfonamides can produce severe, possibly fatal, reactions such as toxic epidermal necrolysis and Stevens–Johnson syndrome

Reactions

Skin

Angioedema
Dermatitis (eyedrops) [6]
Diaphoresis
Eczema [2]
Edema (0.6%)
Erythema multiforme
Erythroderma [2]
Exanthems
Exfoliative dermatitis
Hyperkeratosis (palms and soles)
Lichenoid eruption [1]
Lupus erythematosus [2]
Pemphigus [1]
Photosensitivity
Pigmentation
Pityriasis rubra pilaris [1]
Pruritus (1–5%) [1]
Psoriasis [5]
Purpura
Rash (sic) (1–10%)
Raynaud's phenomenon [2]
Toxic epidermal necrolysis
Urticaria
Xerosis

Hair

Hair – alopecia (1–10%) [2]

Nails

Nails – dystrophy
Nails – onycholysis
Nails – pigmentation [1]

Eyes

Conjunctivitis [1]
Eyelid dermatitis [3]
Ocular allergy [2]
Ocular burning [4]
Ocular lichenoid eruption [1]
Ocular pemphigoid [1]
Ocular stinging [5]
Oculo-mucocutaneous syndrome [1]

Other

Anaphylactoid reactions
Digital necrosis [1]
Dysgeusia
Headache
Myalgia
Oral lichenoid eruption
Paresthesias (<1%)
Peyronie's disease [1]
Tinnitus
Xerostomia (19%) [3]

Note: Cutaneous side-effects of beta-receptor blockaders are clinically polymorphous. They apparently appear after several months of continuous therapy. Atypical psoriasiform, lichen planus-like, and eczematous chronic rashes are mainly observed. (1983): Hödl St, *Z Hautkr* (German) 1:58, 17

TINZAPARIN

Trade name: Innohep (Pharmion)
Indications: Acute symptomatic deep vein thrombosis
Category: Anticoagulant; Low-molecular weight heparin; Thrombolytic
Half-life: 3–4 hours
Clinically important, potentially hazardous interactions with: butabarbital

Reactions

Skin
Abscess (<1%)
Allergic reactions (sic)
Angioedema (<1%)
Bullous eruption (1–10%)
Cellulitis (<1%)
Exanthems (<1%)
Infections
Necrosis (1%)
Neoplasms
Pruritus (1–10%)
Purpura (<1%) [1]
Rash (sic) (1%)
Urticaria (<1%)

Hair
Hair – alopecia [1]

Hematopoietic
Ecchymoses

Other
Anaphylactoid reactions (In sulfite-sensitive people)
Headache
Hypersensitivity
Injection-site bleeding [1]
Injection-site hematoma (16%)
Injection-site pain
Phlebitis
Priapism (<1%) [1]
Thrombophlebitis

TIROFIBAN

Trade name: Aggrastat (Merck)
Indications: Acute coronary syndrome
Category: Platelet aggregation inhibitor
Half-life: 2 hours
Clinically important, potentially hazardous interactions with: aspirin, fondaparinux, heparin

Reactions

Skin
Bleeding
Diaphoresis (2%)
Edema (2%)
Rash (sic) (<1%)
Urticaria (<1%)

Other
Limb pain (3%)

TIZANIDINE

Trade name: Zanaflex (Acorda)
Other common trade names: *Sirdalud; Ternalax; Ternelin*
Indications: Muscle spasticity, multiple sclerosis
Category: Alpha-2-adrenoceptor blocker
Half-life: 2.5 hours

Reactions

Skin
Acne (<1%)
Allergic reactions (sic) (<1%)
Candidiasis (<1%)
Cellulitis (<1%)
Diaphoresis (>1%)
Edema (<1%)
Exanthems (<1%)
Exfoliative dermatitis (<1%)
Herpes simplex (<1%)
Herpes zoster (<1%)
Petechiae (<1%)
Pruritus (1–10%)
Purpura (<1%)
Rash (sic) (1–10%)
Ulcerations (>1%)
Urticaria (<1%)
Xerosis (<1%)

Hair
Hair – alopecia (<1%)

Hematopoietic
Ecchymoses (<1%)

Other
Paresthesias (>1%)
Tremor (1–10%)
Vulvovaginal candidiasis (<1%)
Xerostomia (49%)

TOCAINIDE

Trade name: Tonocard (AstraZeneca)
Indications: Ventricular arrhythmias
Category: Antiarrhythmic class I B
Half-life: 11–14 hours

Reactions

Skin
Allergic reactions (sic) [2]
Clammy skin
Diaphoresis (<1%)
Erythema multiforme (<1%)
Exanthems [1]
Exfoliative dermatitis (<1%)
Lupus erythematosus (<1%) [2]
Pallor (<1%)
Pruritus (<1%)
Rash (sic) (0.5–8.4%)
Stevens–Johnson syndrome (<1%)
Vasculitis (<1%)

Hair
Hair – alopecia (<1%)

Other
Dysgeusia (8.4%)
Gingivitis [1]
Headache

Hypersensitivity (<1%)
Myalgia (<1%)
Paresthesias (3.5–9%)
Parosmia (<1%)
Stomatitis (<1%)
Tinnitus
Xerostomia (<1%)

TOLAZAMIDE*

Trade name: Tolinase (Pfizer)
Other common trade names: *Diabewas; Diadutos; Norglycin; Tolanase; Tolisan*
Indications: Non-insulin dependent diabetes type II
Category: First generation sulfonylurea hypoglycemic
Half-life: 7 hours

Reactions

Skin
Dermatitis [1]
Diaphoresis
Eczema [1]
Erythema (0.4%)
Exanthems (0.4%)
Lichenoid eruption [2]
Lupus erythematosus
Photosensitivity (1–10%)
Pruritus (0.4%)
Purpura
Rash (sic) (1–10%)
Urticaria (1–10%)

Other
Acute intermittent porphyria
Dysgeusia
Paresthesias
Porphyria cutanea tarda
Tongue ulceration [1]

***Note:** Tolazamide is a sulfonamide and can be absorbed systemically. Sulfonamides can produce severe, possibly fatal, reactions such as toxic epidermal necrolysis and Stevens–Johnson syndrome

TOLAZOLINE

Trade name: Priscoline (Novartis)
Indications: Pulmonary hypertension in the newborn
Category: Alpha-adrenoceptor blocker; Antihypertensive (of the newborn); Peripheral vasodilator
Half-life: 3–10 hours (neonates)

Reactions

Skin
Dermatitis [1]
Edema
Exanthems [1]
Flushing (66%) [1]
Rash (sic)
Urticaria

Other
Injection-site burning (>10%)

TOLBUTAMIDE*

Trade name: Orinase (Pfizer)
Other common trade names: *Abemin; Aglycid; Diaben; Diatol; Dolipol; Mobenol; Novo-Butamid; Orabet; Rastinon*
Indications: Non-insulin dependent diabetes type II
Category: First generation sulfonylurea hypoglycemic
Half-life: 4–25 hours
Clinically important, potentially hazardous interactions with: aprepitant

Reactions

Skin
- Allergic reactions (sic) (<1%) [1]
- Bullous eruption (<1%)
- Bullous pemphigoid [1]
- Dermatitis [1]
- Erythema (1.1%)
- Erythema multiforme (<1%)
- Exanthems (1–5%) [3]
- Fixed eruption (<1%)
- Flushing [3]
- Lichenoid eruption [1]
- Photosensitivity (1–10%) [2]
- Poikiloderma [1]
- Pruritus (1.1%)
- Purpura [2]
- Rash (sic) (1–10%)
- Side effects (sic) (1%) [3]
- Toxic epidermal necrolysis (<1%)
- Urticaria (1–10%) [1]

Other
- Acute intermittent porphyria
- Disulfiram-like reaction
- Dysgeusia
- Headache
- Hypersensitivity (<1%)
- Injection-site thrombophlebitis (<1%)
- Oral lichenoid eruption
- Paresthesias
- Porphyria [1]
- Porphyria cutanea tarda [1]
- Thrombophlebitis (<1%)

***Note:** Tolbutamide is a sulfonamide and can be absorbed systemically. Sulfonamides can produce severe, possibly fatal, reactions such as toxic epidermal necrolysis and Stevens–Johnson syndrome

TORSEMIDE*

Trade name: Demadex (Roche)
Other common trade name: *Unat*
Indications: Edema
Category: Antihypertensive; Sulfonylurea loop diuretic
Half-life: 2–4 hours
Clinically important, potentially hazardous interactions with: amikacin, gentamicin, kanamycin, neomycin, streptomycin, tobramycin

Reactions

Skin

- Angioedema
- Edema (1.1%)
- Exanthems
- Lichenoid eruption [1]
- Photosensitivity (1–10%)
- Pruritus
- Purpura [1]
- Rash (sic) (<1%)
- Stevens–Johnson syndrome [1]
- Urticaria (1–10%)
- Vasculitis [2]

Other

- Headache
- Injection-site erythema (<1%)
- Myalgia (1.6%)
- Tinnitus
- Xerostomia

***Note:** Torsemide is a sulfonamide and can be absorbed systemically. Sulfonamides can produce severe, possibly fatal, reactions such as toxic epidermal necrolysis and Stevens–Johnson syndrome

TRANDOLAPRIL

Trade names: Mavik (Abbott); Tarka (Abbott)
Other common trade names: *Gopten; Odrik; Udrik*
Indications: Hypertension
Category: Angiotensin-converting enzyme (ACE) inhibitor; Antihypertensive; Calcium channel blocker (with verapamil)
Half-life: 24 hours
Clinically important, potentially hazardous interactions with: amiloride, spironolactone, triamterene

Tarka is trandolapril and verapamil

Reactions

Skin

- Angioedema (0.15%) [2]
- Edema (>3%)
- Flushing (>3%)
- Pemphigus (<1%)
- Pemphigus foliaceus [1]
- Pruritus (>3%)
- Rash (sic) (>10%)

Other

- Cough [2]
- Headache
- Hyperesthesia (>3%)
- Myalgia (>3%)
- Paresthesias (>3%)
- Rhabdomyolysis [1]
- Xerostomia (>3%)

TREPROSTINIL

Trade name: Remodulin (United)
Indications: Pulmonary arterial hypertension
Category: Platelet Inhibitor; Prostaglandin; Vasodilator
Half-life: 2–4 hours

Reactions

Skin
- Diaphoresis
- Edema (9%)
- Erythema
- Flushing
- Peripheral edema
- Pruritus (8%)
- Rash (sic) (14%)

Other
- Application-site reactions (sic) (83%)
- Dizziness (9%)
- Headache (27%)
- Injection-site bleeding (33%)
- Injection-site induration
- Injection-site pain (85%) [2]
- Injection-site reactions (sic) (83%)
- Pain (13%)
- Pharyngitis (12%)

TRIAMTERENE

Trade names: Dyazide (GSK); Dyrenium (Wellspring); Maxzide (Mylan Bertek)
Other common trade names: *Amterene; Diarrol; Diuteren; Dytac; Reviten; Suloton; Trian*
Indications: Edema
Category: Antihypertensive; Potassium-sparing antihypertensive diuretic
Half-life: 1–2 hours
Clinically important, potentially hazardous interactions with: benazepril, captopril, cyclosporine, enalapril, fosinopril, indomethacin, **juniper**, lisinopril, moexipril, potassium iodide, quinapril, ramipril, spironolactone, trandolapril

Dyazide is triamterene and hydrochlorothiazide*; Maxzide is triamterene and hydrochlorothiazide*

Reactions

Skin
- Chills
- Diaphoresis [1]
- Edema (1–10%)
- Exanthems
- Flushing (<1%)
- Lupus erythematosus (with hydrochlorothiazide) [2]
- Perleche
- Photosensitivity [2]
- Pruritus
- Purpura
- Rash (sic) (1–10%)
- Urticaria
- Vasculitis

Other
- Anaphylactoid reactions
- Dysgeusia [1]

Glossitis
Gynecomastia (<1%)
Headache
Paresthesias
Pseudoporphyria [1]
Stomatodynia [1]
Xerostomia [1]

***Note:** Hydrochlorothiazide is a sulfonamide and can be absorbed systemically. Sulfonamides can produce severe, possibly fatal, reactions such as toxic epidermal necrolysis and Stevens–Johnson syndrome

TRICHLORMETHIAZIDE*

Trade name: Naqua
Other common trade names: *Anatran; Aquacot; Carvacron; Diurese; Doqua; Esmarin; Flute; Iopran; Niazide; Trichlon; Trichlorex*
Indications: Edema, hypertension
Category: Antihypertensive; Thiazide diuretic
Half-life: N/A
Clinically important, potentially hazardous interactions with: digoxin, lithium

Reactions

Skin
Exanthems
Lichenoid eruption (<1%)
Lupus erythematosus [1]
Photosensitivity (<1%)
Purpura [1]
Rash (sic)
Urticaria
Vasculitis [1]

Other
Anaphylactoid reactions
Paresthesias
Xerostomia

***Note:** Trichlormethiazide is a sulfonamide and can be absorbed systemically. Sulfonamides can produce severe, possibly fatal, reactions such as toxic epidermal necrolysis and Stevens–Johnson syndrome

UROKINASE

Trade name: Abbokinase (Abbott)
Other common trade name: *Ukidan*
Indications: Acute myocardial infarction, coronary artery thrombosis, pulmonary embolism
Category: Thrombolytic enzyme
Half-life: 10–20 minutes
Clinically important, potentially hazardous interactions with: aspirin, bivalirudin, ibuprofen, indomethacin

Reactions

Skin
- Angioedema (>10%) [1]
- Bleeding (44%)
- Bullous eruption (hemorrhagic) [1]
- Chills
- Diaphoresis (<1%)
- Exanthems
- Flushing
- Pruritus
- Purpura
- Rash (sic) (<1%)
- Urticaria

Eyes
- Periorbital edema (>10%)

Hematopoietic
- Ecchymoses

Other
- Anaphylactoid reactions (>10%) [1]
- Hypersensitivity [1]
- Injection-site phlebitis

VALSARTAN

Trade name: Diovan (Novartis)
Indications: Hypertension
Category: Angiotensin II receptor antagonist; Antihypertensive
Half-life: 9 hours

Reactions

Skin
- Allergic reactions (sic) (>2%)
- Angioedema (>2%) [2]
- Edema (>1%) [2]
- Flushing [1]
- Photosensitivity [1]
- Pruritus (>2%)
- Rash (sic) (>2%)
- Urticaria [1]

Nails
- Nails – onychocryptosis
- Nails – pigmentation

Other
- Aphthous stomatitis (1–10%)
- Arthralgia (1–10%)
- Cough [1]
- Death [1]
- Depression [1]
- Dysgeusia (>10%)
- Headache
- Injection-site extravasation (<1%)
- Injection-site pain
- Injection-site phlebitis
- Injection-site reactions (sic)
- Myalgia (10–29%)
- Paresthesias (>2%)
- Xerostomia (>10%)

VERAPAMIL

Trade names: Calan (Pfizer); Covera-HS (Pfizer); Isoptin (Abbott); Tarka (Abbott); Verelan (Schwarz)

Other common trade names: *APO-Verap; Arpamyl LP; Azupamil; Berkatens; Chronovera; Cordilox; Geangin; Isoptine; Nu-Verap; Veraken*

Indications: Angina, hypertension

Category: Antianginal; Antihypertensive; Calcium channel blocker

Half-life: 2–8 hours

Clinically important, potentially hazardous interactions with: acebutolol, amiodarone, aspirin, atenolol, atorvastatin, betaxolol, carbamazepine, carteolol, clonidine, dantrolene, digoxin, dofetilide, epirubicin, eplerenone, erythromycin, esmolol, **eucalyptus**, lovastatin, metoprolol, **mistletoe**, nadolol, penbutolol, pindolol, propranolol, quinidine, sibutramine, simvastatin, telithromycin, timolol

Tarka is trandolapril and verapamil

Reactions

Skin
- Acne [1]
- Acute febrile neutrophilic dermatosis (Sweet's syndrome) [1]
- Angioedema [3]
- Dermatitis
- Diaphoresis (<1%) [2]
- Edema (1.9%)
- Erythema multiforme (<1%) [4]
- Erythema nodosum [1]
- Exanthems [7]
- Exfoliative dermatitis [2]
- Flushing (1–7%) [4]
- Hyperkeratosis (palms) (<1%) [2]
- Lichenoid eruption
- Lupus erythematosus [2]
- Peripheral edema (1–10%) [1]
- Photosensitivity [4]
- Prurigo [1]
- Pruritus [6]
- Purpura (<1%) [1]
- Rash (sic) (1.2%) [2]
- Side effects (sic) [2]
- Stevens–Johnson syndrome (<1%) [4]
- Urticaria (<1%) [5]
- Vasculitis (<1%) [2]

Hair
- Hair – alopecia (<1%) [6]
- Hair – hypertrichosis [1]
- Hair – pigmentation [1]

Nails
- Nails – dystrophy [1]

Hematopoietic
- Ecchymoses (<1%) [1]

Other
- Erythromelalgia [1]
- Galactorrhea (<1%)
- Gingival hypertrophy (19%) [4]
- Gynecomastia (<1%) [4]
- Headache
- Paresthesias (<1%)
- Parkinsonism [1]
- Rhabdomyolysis [1]
- Serum sickness [1]
- Xerostomia (<1%)

WARFARIN

Trade name: Coumadin (Bristol-Myers Squibb)
Other common trade names: *Aldocumar; Coumadine; Marevan; Waran; Warfilone*
Indications: Thromboembolic disease, pulmonary embolism
Category: Anticoagulant
Half-life: 1.5–2.5 days (highly variable)
Clinically important, potentially hazardous interactions with: amiodarone, amobarbital, aprepitant, aprobarbital, **arnica**, aspirin, azathioprine, azithromycin, bismuth, bivalirudin, bosentan, butabarbital, **capsicum**, **chamomile**, cimetidine, clarithromycin, clarithromycin, clofibrate, clopidogrel, clorazepate, co trimoxazole, **coenzyme Q-10**, cyclosporine, **dan-shen**, danazol, daptomycin, delavirdine, **devil's claw**, dirithromycin, disulfiram, **dong quai**, erythromycin, **evening Primrose**, fenofibrate, **feverfew**, fluconazole, fluoxymesterone, fosamprenavir, **garlic**, gemfibrozil, **ginger**, **ginkgo biloba**, **ginseng**, glucagon, **grapefruit Juice**, **green tea**, **guarana**, **horse chestnut (bark, flower, leaf, seed**, imatinib, **influenza Vaccines**, itraconazole, itraconazole, ketoconazole, levothyroxine, liothyronine, **melatonin**, mephobarbital, methimazole, methyltestosterone, metronidazole, miconazole, nalidixic acid, peg interferon alfa-2b, penicillins, pentobarbital, phenobarbital, phenobarbital, phytonadione, piperacillin, primidone, propoxyphene, propylthiouracil, quinidine, quinine, **red clover**, rifampin, rifapentine, rifapentine, rofecoxib, rosuvastatin, **saw palmetto**, secobarbital, **st john's wort**, stanozolol, sulfamethoxazole, sulfinpyrazone, sulfisoxazole, sulindac, testosterone, troleandomycin, troleandomycin, valdecoxib, vitamin A, vitamin E, zileuton

Note: Alternative remedies, including herbals, may potentially increase the risk of bleeding or potentiate the effects of warfarin therapy. Some of these include the following: angelica root, arnica flower, anise, asafetida, bogbean, borage seed oil, bromelain, dan shen, devil's claw, fenugreek, feverfew, garlic, ginger, ginkgo biloba, ginseng, horse chestnut, lovage root, meadowsweet, onion, parsley, passionflower herb, poplar, quassia, red clover, rue, turmeric and willow bark

Reactions

Skin

Abscess [1]
Acral purpura [1]
Angioedema (<1%)
Bullous eruption [2]
Dermatitis [2]
Exanthems [7]
Exfoliative dermatitis
Hematomas [1]
Hemorrhage [3]
Lingual hemorrhage [1]
Livedo reticularis [1]
Necrosis (>10%) [85]
Pruritus (<1%) [2]
Purple toe syndrome [1]
Purplish erythema (feet and toes) (<1%) [8]
Purpura [3]
Rash (sic) (<1%) [1]
Ulcerations [1]
Urticaria [3]
Vasculitis [4]
Vesiculation [1]

Hair

Hair – alopecia (>10%) [6]

Hematopoietic
Ecchymoses [2]

Other
Death [1]

Gangrene [3]
Hypersensitivity [2]
Oral ulceration (<1%)
Priapism [2]

YOHIMBINE

Scientific name: *Pausinystalia yohimbe*
Family: Rubiaceae
Trade and other common names: Actibane (Consolidated Midland); Aphrodyne (Star); Yocon (Palisades); Yohimex (Kramer); Yomax
Category: Anesthetic; Aphrodisiac (purported)
Purported indications and other uses: Impotence, alpha2-adrenergic blocker, orthostatic hypertension
Half-life: 36 minutes

Reactions

Skin
Adverse effects (sic) [1]
Diaphoresis
Exfoliative dermatitis [1]
Flushing
Lupus erythematosus [1]

Other
Death

DRUGS RESPONSIBLE FOR COMMON CARDIAC REACTIONS

ANGINA

Albuterol
Alcohol
Alemtuzumab
Apomorphine
Bicalutamide
Blue cohosh
Candesartan
Capecitabine (<5%)
Capsicum
Captopril
Carvedilol (2–6%)
Cevimeline (<1%)
Ciprofloxacin
Clozapine (1–10%)
Cocaine
Diclofenac
Dipyridamole
Dobutamine (1–3%)
Dopamine
Eletriptan (<1%)
Epinephrine
Eprosartan (<1%)
Ergonovine
Felodipine (<1%)
Fenoldopam
Flecainide
Fluorouracil
Fluoxetine (<1%)
Fluvoxamine (<1%)
Fosinopril (<1%)
Gabapentin (<1%)
Granisetron (<1%)
Haloperidol
Halothane
Indomethacin
Interferon alfa 2-b (<5%)
Isosorbide dinitrate
Isosorbide mononitrate (<1%)
Lamotrigine (<1%)
Lansoprazole (<1%)
Latanoprost
Letrozole (<2%)
Leuprolide
Levothyroxine
Marihuana
Meloxicam (<1%)
Metaproterenol (<1%)
Metaraminol
Methamphetamine
Methylphenidate
Mexiletine (2%)
Minoxidil (<1%)
Mycophenolate (3%)
Nabumetone (<1%)
Nesiritide (2%)
Nicardipine
Nifedipine
Nitroglycerin (2%)
Omeprazole (<1%)
Ondansetron (<1%)
Oral contraceptives
Oseltamivir (<1%)
Pantoprazole (<1%)
Pilocarpine (<1%)
Prazosin (<1%)
Progesterone (<5%)
Propafenone (<3%)
Quinapril (<1%)
Quinidine (6%)
Quinine
Quinupristin/Dalfopristin (<1%)
Ramipril (3%)
Rosuvastatin (1%)
Selegiline
Sibutramine
Sildenafil (<2%)
Sparfloxacin (<1%)
Sumatriptan (<1%)
Tacrolimus (3–15%)

Tadalafil (<2%)
Tegaserod (1–10%)
Telmisartan (<1%)
Timolol (<1%)
Tinzaparin (1–10%)
Tocainide (1%)
Toremifene (1–10%)
Trandolapril (<1%)
Travoprost (1–5%
Valdecoxib (<2%)
Vardenafil (<2%)
Verapamil (<1%)
Zalcitabine (<1%)
Zaleplon (<1%)
Ziprasidone (<1%)

ARRHYTHMIAS

Adalimumab
Adenosine
Aldesleukin
Amifostine
Amiloride
Aminocaproic acid (1–10%)
Amiodarone (<3%)
Amitriptyline
Amlodipine (<1%)
Angiotensin inhibitors
Antiarrhythmics class 1C
Antidepressants
Arsenic
Astemizole
Atenolol
Atorvastatin (<2%)
Atropine
Azithromycin (<1%)
Beta-blockers
Bortezomib
Bromocriptine
Bupropion (1–10%)
Caffeine
Calcium channel blockers
Carbamazepine
Carmustine
Carteolol (<1%)
Cevimeline (<1%)
Chloroquine
Chlorpromazine
Cilostazol (<2%)
Cisplatin
Clofibrate
Clozapine
Cocaine
Codeine (1–10%)
Cyclobenzaprine (<1%)
Cycloserine
Cyclosporine (1–10%)
Daptomycin (<1%)
Denileukin (6%)
Desipramine
Diclofenac
Diflunisal (1–10%)
Digoxin
Diltiazem (<2%)
Dinoprostone (<1%)
Dipyridamole (<1%)
Dirithromycin (<1%)
Disopyramide
Diuretics
Docetaxel (<1%)
Dopamine
Doxazosin (2%)
Doxorubicin (1–10%)
Droperidol (<1%)
Edrophonium
Eletriptan (<1%)
Ephedra
Ephedrine
Epinephrine
Erythromycin
Estrogens
Etodolac (<1%)
Felodipine (<1%)
Fenofibrate
Fenoprofen (<1%)
Fentanyl (1–10%)
Fluoxetine (<1%)
Fluphenazine
Foscarnet (<1%)

Gadodiamide
Ganciclovir (<1%)
Haloperidol
Hydralazine
Inamrinone (3%)
Indomethacin (<1%)
Infliximab (<2%)
Interferon alfa 2-b (<5%)
Interferon beta-1b (<1%)
Irbesartan (<1%)
Isosorbide mononitrate (<1%)
Itraconazole (<1%)
Ketamine (<1%)
Lansoprazole (<1%)
Leuprolide
Levalbuterol (<2%)
Levodopa
Levofloxacin (<1%)
Levothyroxine
Lidocaine
Lindane
Lisinopril (<1%)
Lithium
Lomefloxacin (<1%)
Loratadine
Losartan (<1%)
Loxapine
Macrolide antibiotics
Meclofenamate (<1%)
Mefenamic acid
Meloxicam (<1%)
Meprobamate (<1%)
Meropenem (<1%)
Metaraminol
Methadone
Methylphenidate
Metoprolol (<1%)
Milrinone (~10%)
Misoprostol (<1%)
Mitoxantrone (3–18%)
Modafinil (1%)
Moexipril (<1%)
Molindone
Moricizine (<1%)
Mycophenolate (3–20%)
Nabumetone (<1%)
Nadolol (<1%)
Naloxone
Naproxen (<1%)
Neostigmine
Niacin
Nortriptyline
Octreotide (3–9%)
Oseltamivir (<1%)
Oxybutynin
Palonosetron (<1%)
Pantoprazole (<1%)
Peg-interferon alfa-2a (<1%)
Peg-interferon alfa-2b (<1%)
Pentamidine (1–10%)
Pentostatin (1–10%)
Pentoxifylline (<1%)
Pergolide (1%)
Phenothiazines
Phentolamine
Phenylephrine
Phenytoin
Pilocarpine (<1%)
Pimozide
Pirbuterol (<1%)
Primaquine
Procainamide
Propafenone (2–10%)
Propofol (1–3%)
Propranolol
Protriptylin
Pseudoephedrine
Pyridostigmine
Pyrimethamine
Quinapril (<1%)
Quinidine (1–10%)
Quinupristin/Dalfopristin (<1%)
Ramipril (<1%)
Ranitidine
Rituximab (<1%)
Sotalol
Tacrolimus
Terfenadine

Theophylline
Thioridazine
Timolol
Warfarin
Ziprasidone

ATRIAL FIBRILLATION

Acetylcholine
Adalimumab
Adenosine
Albuterol
Alcohol
Amifostine
Aminophylline
Amiodarone
Amphotericin B
Anagrelide
Apomorphine
Arbutamine
Argatroban (3%)
Aripiprazole (<1%)
Atenolol
Atropine (1–10%)
Azathioprine
Bupivacaine
Caffeine
Cisplatin
Clopidogrel
Clozapine
Dexmedetomidine (7%)
Digoxin
Diltiazem
Disopyramide
Disulfiram
Dobutamine
Docetaxel (<1%)
Donepezil (1–10%)
Dopamine
Dopexamine
Etanercept
Etoposide
Etretinate
Fenofibrate
Flosequinan
Fluorouracil
Fluoxetine
Galantamine
Gemcitabine
Granisetron (<1%)
Ifosfamide
Interferon alfa-2b (<5%)
Interferon gamma
Interleukins 3, 6
Isosorbide mononitrate
Isradipine
Losartan
Melphalan
Methylprednisolone (high dose)
Naratriptan
Nesiritide (1–10%)
Niacin
Nicotine
Pamidronate (<6%)
Paroxetine (<1%)
Pentagastrin
Perflexane
Perfluorobutane
Physostigmine
Porfimer
Propafenone (1%)
Pseudoephedrine
Sildenafil
Sumatriptan
Terbutaline
Thiazides
Tranylcypromine
Trazodone
Verapamil
Verteporfin
Zalcitabine

ATRIOVENTRICULAR BLOCK (A-V BLOCK)

Abciximab (<1%)
Alteplase
Amiodarone (5%)
Aripiprazole (<1%)
Atenolol (1–10%)

Bupropion
Carbamazepine
Carvedilol (3%)
Clonidine (<1%)
Diltiazem (<2%)
Dipyridamole (<1%)
Disopyramide (<1%)
Dofetilide (1%)
Edrophonium
Flecainide (<1%)
Ibutilide (2%)
Losartan (<1%)
Mefloquine (<1%)
Metoclopramide (<1%)
Mexiletine (<1%)
Nefazodone (<1%)
Nisoldipine (<1%)
Pergolide (<1%)
Propafenone (<1%)
Pyridostigmine
Sertraline (<1%)
Sildenafil (<2%)
Sparfloxacin (<1%)
Streptokinase
Tenecteplase
Tocainide (<1%)
Topiramate (<1%)
Trandolapril (<1%)

BRADYCARDIA

Acebutolol (1–10%)
Adenosine
Alfentanil
Alprostadil
Alteplase
Aminocaproic acid
Amiodarone
Amlodipine (<1%)
Aprepitant
Aripiprazole (1%)
Atenolol
Atracurium (<1%)
Atropine
Bepridil (1–10%)
Beta-blockers
Betaxolol (1–10%)
Bisoprolol (1–10%)
Bivalirudin (1–10%)
Bupivacaine
Buprenorphine (<1%)
Calcium channel blockers
Carbamazepine
Carteolol
Carvedilol (2–10%)
Cimetidine (<1%)
Cisatracurium
Cisplatin (<1%)
Citalopram
Clomipramine
Clonidine (<1%)
Cocaine (1–10%)
Dexmedetomidine (1–10%)
Digoxin
Diltiazem (2–6%)
Dinoprostone (1–10%)
Dipyridamole (<1%)
Dopamine
Doxercalciferol (7%)
Edrophonium
Esmolol (<1%)
Estrogens
Etidocaine
Etomidate (<1%)
Famotidine (<1%)
Fentanyl (>10%)
Flecainide
Fluoxetine
Fluvoxamine (<1%)
Fomepizole (<1%)
Foscarnet (<1%)
Fosphenytoin (<1%)
Frovatriptan (<1%)
Galantamine (2–3%)
Ginger
Hydromorphone
Ibutilide (1%)
Imipramine
Infliximab (<2%)

Irinotecan
Isoproterenol
Isosorbide dinitrate
Ivabradin
Ketamine
Labetalol
Levofloxacin (<1%)
Levorphanol
Lidocaine
Lithium
Lopinavir
Lorazepam
Marihuana
Mefloquine (<1%)
Mepivicaine
Methadone
Metoprolol
Mistletoe
Morphine
Nadolol (1–10%)
Nalbuphine (<1%)
Nefazodone (1–10%)
Neostigmine
Nimodipine
Nitroglycerin
Octreotide (19–25%)
Oxprenolol
Paclitaxel
Palonosetron (1%)
Pentazocine
Perflutren (<0.5%)
Perphenazine
Phenformin
Phenobarbital
Phenylephrine
Phenytoin
Physostigmine
Pindolol (<1%)
Pirezepine
Prochlorperazine
Promethazine
Propafenone (1–2%)
Propofol (1–3%)
Propranolol
Protamine
Protamine sulfate
Pyridostigmine
Quinidine (<1%)
Rabeprazole
Remifentanil (1–10%)
Reserpine
Ritonavir
Rue
Sotalol
Succinylcholine
Sulprostone
Tacrine
Timolol
Tocainide
Trazodone
Verapamil
Voriconazole

CARDIAC (HEART) FAILURE

Alteplase
Amlodipine (<1%)
Aprotinin (1–10%)
Atenolol (1–10%)
Capecitabine (<5%)
Clopidogrel (1–3%)
Cyclophosphamide
Cyclosporine (1–10%)
Ertapenem (<1%)
Etanercept (<3%)
Foscarnet (<1%)
Galantamine (<1%)
Infliximab (<2%)
Interferon beta-1b (<1%)
Irbesartan (<1%)
Isradipine (<1%)
Levothyroxine
Meloxicam (<2%)
Memantine (1–10%)
Meropenem (<1%)
Mycophenolate (3–20%)
Oxcarbazepine (<1%)
Pamidronate (~1%)
Porfimer (1–10%)

Rivastigmine (<2%)
Ropinirole (<1%)
Sildenafil (<2%)
Streptokinase
Toremifene (1–10%)
Tretinoin (1–10%)

CARDIOMYOPATHY

Amiodarone (<5%)
Capecitabine (<5%)
Chloroquine
Clozapine (<1%)
Cocaine (1–10%)
Glatiramer (<1%)
Hydroxychloroquine
Interferon alfa-2a (<1%)
Interferon alfa-2b (<5%)
Interferon beta-1a (<1%)
Megestrol
Sildenafil (<2%)
Tretinoin (1-10%)

CARDIAC ARREST

Adalimumab (<5%)
Alemtuzumab (<1%)
Alprostadil (1–10%)
Alteplase
Amifostine (<1%)
Amiodarone (1–10%)
Amphotericin B (<1%)
Argatroban (6%)
Atazanavir (<3%)
Bortezomib (<1%)
Bupivacaine
Capecitabine (<5%)
Cilostazol (<2%)
Daclizumab (<1%)
Dofetilide (<2%)
Edrophonium
Ephedra
Ertapenem (<2%)
Estramustine (<1%)
Flucytosine
Furosemide
Infliximab (<2%)
Interferon beta-1b (<1%)
Levothyroxine
Lisinopril (<1%)
Methadone
Mistletoe
Moxifloxacin (<3%)
Perphenazine
Propafenone (<1%)
Propofol (<1%)
Pyridostigmine
Quinupristin/Dalfopristin (<1%)
Rivastigmine (<2%)
Ropinirole (<1%)
Sildenafil (<2%)
Streptokinase
Tenecteplase
Trastuzumab (<2%)
Tretinoin (1–10%)
Trifluoperazine

CHEST PAIN

Abciximab (10%)
Acamprosate
Acitretin (<1%)
Adalimumab
Adenosine
Agalsidase
Alemtuzumab (10%)
Alfuzosin
Apomorphine
Atorvastatin (2–10%)
Azacitidine
Aztreonam
Betaxolol (<1%)
Bupropion
Cinacalcet
Clofibrate
Clonidine (<1%)
Clopidogrel (8%)
Cocaine
Cromolyn
Cyclosporine (1–10%)
Daclizumab (~5%)

Delavirdine (<1%)
Denileukin (24%)
Desmopressin
Diflunisal (1–10%)
Dirithromycin (1–10%)
Dobutamine (1–3%)
Dofetilide (10%)
Donepezil (1–10%)
Dornase alfa
Doxazosin (1–2%)
Doxorubicin
Eletriptan (1–10%)
Enalapril (2%)
Ephedrine
Epinephrine
Epoetin alfa (1–10%)
Ertapenem (<1%)
Escitalopram (1–10%)
Esmolol (<1%)
Exemestane (1–10%)
Ezetimibe (3%)
Felbamate (1–10%)
Fenoldopam
Filgrastim (1–10%)
Flecainide (5%)
Flucytosine
Fluorides
Fluorouracil (<1%)
Fluoxetine (<1%)
Frovatriptan (2%)
Fulvestrant (7%)
Galantamine (1)
Gatifloxacin (<3%)
Glatiramer (21%)
Goserelin (1–10%)
Haloperidol
Imiglucerase
Inamrinone (<1%)
Infliximab
Interferon alfa-2b (2–28%)
Interferon alfa-2a (4–11%)
Interferon beta-1a (1–10%)
Interferon beta-1b (1–10%)
Isoproterenol
Isotretinoin
Isradipine (<2%)
Lansoprazole (<1%)
Laronidase (9%)
Leflunomide (2%)
Letrozole (3–8%)
Levetiracetam (1–10%)
Levodopa
Levorphanol
Lomefloxacin (<1%)
Loratadine (<2%)
Losartan (12%)
Marihuana
Mefloquine (<1%)
Mesalamine (3%)
Metaproterenol (<1%)
Metolazone (1–10%)
Metoprolol (<1%)
Mexiletine (3–8%)
Milrinone (<1%)
Modafinil (2%)
Moexipril (<1%)
Monosodium glutamate
Moricizine (<1%)
Moxifloxacin (<3%)
Mycophenolate (3–20%)
Nadolol (<1%)
Nafarelin (1–10%)
Naloxone
Nedocromil (1–10%)
Neostigmine
Nicotine (1%)
Nimodipine (2%)
Nitrofurantoin
Olanzapine (1–10%)
Olmesartan (<1%)
Ondansetron (<1%)
Oxaliplatin
Pantoprazole (~6%)
Peg-interferon alfa-2a (<1%)
Pegvisomant (4–8%)
Pemetrexed
Pentamidine (>10%)
Pentostatin (1–10%)

Pentoxifylline (<1%)
Perflutren
Perindopril (2%)
Pindolol (3%)
Pirbuterol (<1%)
Piroxicam (<1%)
Pramipexole (1–10%)
Pravastatin (4%)
Prochlorperazine
Progesterone (<5%)
Propafenone (1–2%)
Propranolol
Quinapril (2%)
Raloxifene (1–10%)
Rasburicase
Repaglinide (2–3%)
Ribavirin
Rifabutin (<1%)
Rifaximin
Risedronate
Tiotropium
Tositumomab & Iodine131
Verteporfin

CONGESTIVE HEART FAILURE

Adriamycin
Amitriptyline
Ampicillin
Anesthetics
Apomorphine (>5%)
Beta-blockers
Betaxolol (1–10%)
Bicalutamide
Bisoprolol
Bortezomib
Buspirone
Captopril
Carbamazepine
Carteolol (1–10%)
Carvedilol
Celecoxib (<2%)
Cilostazol (<2%)
Clozapine
Cocaine (1–10%)
Cyanocobalamin (<1%)
Cyclophosphamide (<1%)
Cytostatics
Daunomycin
Daunorubicin (1–10%)
Diclofenac (<1%)
Diltiazem (<2%)
Dirithromycin (1–10%)
Donepezil (<1%)
Doxorubicin (1–10%)
Encainide
Epirubicin (<1%)
Esmolol (<1%)
Etanercept (<3%)
Ethmozine
Felodipine (<1%)
Fenoprofen (<1%)
Flecainide (<1%)
Fludarabine (1–10%)
Fluoxetine (<1%)
Flurbiprofen (<1%)
Fosphenytoin (<1%)
Glatiramer (<1%)
Goserelin (5%)
HMG CoA reductase inhibitors
Ibutilide (<1%)
Idarubicin
Imipramine
Indomethacin
Infliximab
Interferon alfa-2b (<5%)
Interleukin 2
Itraconazole
Labetalol (<1%)
Leuprolide
Lorcainide
MDMA
Mefenamic acid (<1%)
Methylxanthines
Metoprolol (<1%)
Mexiletine (<1%)
Minoxidil (>10%)
Mitomycin (3–15%)
Mitoxantrone (2–3%)

Moricizine (1–10%)
Mycophenolate (3–20%)
Nabumetone (<1%)
Nadolol (1–10%)
Naproxen (<1%)
Nimodipine (<1%)
NSAIDs
Oxaliplatin (<1%)
Paclitaxel
Pantoprazole (<1%)
Perphenazine
Phenytoin
Pindolol (<1%)
Pioglitazone (<1%)
Piroxicam (<1%)
Procainamide
Propafenone (1–4%)
Propranolol
Proscillaridin
Quinidine
Spironolactone
Tocainide
Venlafaxine
Verapamil

CORONARY ARTERY DISORDERS

Antiretrovirals
Carbamazepine
Cocaine
Corticosteroids
Cigarette smoking
Granulocyte colony-stimulating factor
Gemcitabine
Heparin
Levodopa
Nicotine
Olanzapine
Protease inhibitors
Sumatriptan

ECG CHANGES (ABNORMALITIES)

Amitriptyline
Aripiprazole
Arsenic trioxide (7%)
Chloroquine
Clozapine (1–10%)
Daunomycin
Dofetilide
Doxorubicin (>10%)
Edrophonium
Escitalopram
Fluorouracil (<1%)
Frovatriptan (<1%)
Hydralazine
Idarubicin (>10%)
Imipramine
Ivermectin
Levalbuterol (<2%)
Lithium
Mitoxantrone (1–10%)
Moricizine (1–10%)
Moxifloxacin (<3%)
Nicardipine (<1%)
Nifedipine
Nimodipine (<1%)
Nitrofurantoin
Ondansetron (<1%)
Pilocarpine (<1%)
Propofol (<1%)
Pyridostigmine
Rocuronium (<1%)
Sumatriptan (<1%)
Tacrolimus (3–15%)
Thioridazine
Thiothixene
Torsemide (2%)

EXTRASYSTOLES

Albuterol
Diltiazem (2%)
Doxorubicin (>10%)
Flumazenil (1–10%)
Fosphenytoin (<1%)
Ibutilide (<1%)
Mefloquine (<1%)
Nesiritide (3%)
Nisoldipine (<1%)

Palonosetron (<1%)
Tizanidine (<1%)

HEART BLOCK

Alprostadil (<1%)
Amitriptyline
Atazanavir (<3%)
Desipramine
Digoxin
Dofetilide (<2%)
Donepezil (<1%)
Doxorubicin (1–10%)
Esmolol (<1%)
Flecainide (<1%)
Imipramine
Labetalol (<1%)
Lidocaine
Meprobamate
Metoprolol (<1%)
Nifedipine
Nortriptyline
Procainamide (<1%)
Protriptyline
Quinidine (<1%)
Sumatriptan (<1%)
Trimipramine

HYPERTENSION

Alcohol
Adrenaline
Alemtuzumab (11%)
Alprostadil (1–10%)
Amitriptyline
Amoxapine
Amphetamines
Amphotericin B (1–10%)
Anastrozole (5–10%)
Aripiprazole (1%)
Atomoxetine (2–9%)
Basiliximab
Bexarotene
Bivalirudin (6%)
Blue cohosh
Bretylium
Buprenorphine
Bupropion
Carvedilol (3%)
Cascara
Caspofungin (2%)
Celecoxib
Cetirizine
Clopidogrel (4%)
Clozapine
Cocaine
Cortisone
Cyclosporine (>10%)
Daclizumab
Daptomycin (1%)
Darbepoetin alfa (4–23%)
Desloratadine
Dipyridamole (2%)
Dobutamine
Dolasetron (3%)
Donepezil (1–10%)
Dopamine
Doxepin
Doxycycline
Droperidol (1–10%)
Ephedrine
Epinephrine
Ergotamine
Ertapenem (1– 2%)
Escitalopram (1–10%)
Esomeprazole (<1%)
Estradiol
Estrogens (conjugated)
Estrogens (esterified)
Ethinyl estradiol
Etodolac (<1%)
Etomidate (<1%)
Exemestane (1–10%)
Famotidine (<1%)
Fenoprofen (<1%)
Fluoxetine (1–10%)
Fluphenazine
Flurbiprofen (<1%)
Flutamide (1%)
Fosphenytoin (<1%)

Gabapentin (<1%)
Gatifloxacin (<3%)
Gemtuzumab (20%)
Ginseng
Glatiramer (1%)
Goserelin (1–10%)
Granisetron (1–2%)
Haloperidol
Hydralazine
Imipramine
Indomethacin (<1%)
Infliximab (10%)
Interferon alfa-2a (11%)
Interferon alfa-2b (9%)
Interferon beta-1b (7%)
Isoproterenol
Ketamine (>10%)
Ketoconazole
Ketorolac (1–10%)
Lamotrigine (<1%)
Laronidase (9%)
Leflunomide (10%)
Leuprolide
Levodopa
Levofloxacin (<1%)
Levothyroxine
Licorice
Linezolid (1–3%)
Lomefloxacin (<1%)
Loxapine
MDMA
Mefenamic acid (<1%)
Megestrol (<1%)
Meloxicam (<2%)
Mesoridazine
Metaproterenol
Metaraminol
Methamphetamine
Methylphenidate
Metoclopramide (<1%)
Midodrine (7%)
Mirtazapine (1–10%)
Moclobemide
Modafinil (2%)
Moricizine (<1%)
Moxifloxacin (<3%)
MSG
Nadolol (<1%)
Naloxone
Nortriptyline
Olanzapine (1–10%)
Oxaliplatin (<1%)
Oxybutynin (2–5%)
Palonosetron (<1%)
Pamidronate (<6%)
Pancuronium
Pegvisomant (4–8%)
Perflutren (<0.5%)
Pergolide (1–10%)
Perphenazine
Phenylephrine
Pilocarpine (3%)
Pirbuterol (<1%)
Piroxicam (<1%)
Prochlorperazine
Progesterone (<5%)
Promethazine
Propofol (8%)
Propranolol
Protriptyline
Remifentanil (1–10%)
Rifapentine (1–10%)
Riluzole (1–10%)
Rivastigmine (3%)
Rizatriptan (1–10%)
Rocuronium (>1%)
Ropinirole (5%)
Rosuvastatin (2–10%)
Salmeterol (<1%)
Selegiline
Sevoflurane (~1%)
Siberian ginseng
Sirolimus (39–49%)
Sodium oxybate (6%)
Solifenacin (0.5–1.4%)
St John's wort
Succinylcholine (<1%)
Sulindac (1%)

Tacrolimus (~15%)
Tadalafil (<2%)
Telmisartan (1%)
Tenecteplase (<1%)
Tinzaparin (1–10%)
Tolcapone (1–10%)
Travoprost (1–5%)
Trazodone (1–10%)
Tretinoin (>10%)
Trimipramine
Unoprostone (1–10%)
Urokinase (<1%)
Valdecoxib (<2%)
Valproic acid (1–10%)
Vardenafil (<2%)
Venlafaxine (3%)
Vinblastine (1–10%)
Vincristine (1–10%)
Voriconazole (2%)
Yohimbine
Zolmitriptan (<1%)

HYPOTENSION

ACE inhibitors
Acebutolol
Acetylcholine
Adenosine
Albuterol
Alcohol
Alfentanil
Alprostadil
Amantadine
Amiodarone
Amlodipine
Argatroban (7%)
Aripiprazole (1%)
Arsenic trioxide (25%)
Asparaginase (<1%)
Atenolol (1–10%)
Atomoxetine (2%)
Atorvastatin (<2%)
Atracurium (<1%)
Atropine
Azithromycin (<1%)
Aztreonam (<1%)
Baclofen
Basiliximab
Benazepril
Bendroflumethiazide
Beta-blockers
Betaxolol
Bethanechol
Bisoprolol
Bivalirudin (12%)
Bloodroot (high doses)
Bosentan (7%)
Bretylium (7%)
Bromocriptine
Bumetanide (<1%)
Bupivacaine
Buprenorphine
Bupropion
Busulfan
Butabarbital
Calcium channel blockers
Captopril (1–2%)
Carbamazepine
Carbidopa
Carmustine
Carteolol
Carvedilol (9–14%)
Caspofungin (1%)
Cefpodoxime
Chlordiazepoxide
Chloroquine
Chlorpromazine
Cidofovir
Cilostazol (<2%)
Cimetidine (<1%)
Cisatracurium
Citalopram
Clemastine
Clindamycin
Clomipramine
Clonidine (3%)
Clorazepate
Clozapine
Codeine

Cyclobenzaprine
Daclizumab (~5%)
Daptomycin (2%)
Darbepoetin alfa (22%)
Deferoxamine
Delavirdine
Denileukin (36%)
Desipramine
Desloratadine
Dexmedetomidine (30%)
Diazepam
Dihydroergotamine
Diltiazem (2–4%)
Dimercaprol (>10%)
Dinoprostone (<1%)
Diphenhydramine
Dipyridamole (5%)
Dirithromycin (1–10%)
Dobutamine
Docetaxel (3%)
Donepezil (1–10%)
Dopamine
Doxacurium
Doxazosin
Doxepin
Dronabinol (1–10%)
Droperidol (1–10%)
Doxazosin
Edrophonium
Enalapril
Enfuvirtide (<1%)
Entacapone (4%)
Ephedrine
Epinephrine
Epoetin alfa (>10%)
Eptifibatide
Ertapenem (1–2%)
Esmolol
Ethionamide
Etomidate (<1%)
Etoposide
Felodipine
Fenoldopam
Fentanyl (>10%)
Fluorouracil (<1%)
Fluoxetine (<1%)
Fluphenazine
Fomepizole (1–10%)
Fondaparinux (4%)
Formoterol (<1%)
Fosphenytoin
Furosemide
Galantamine (<1%)
Gemtuzumab (16%)
Ginseng
Glatiramer (<1%)
Glucagon
Glycopyrrolate (<1%)
Granisetron (<1%)
Guanethidine
Haloperidol
Hepatitis B vaccine
Hydralazine
Hydrochlorothiazide (1–10%)
Hydromorphone
Ibritumomab (6%)
Ibutilide (2%)
Imiglucerase (1–10%)
Imipenem & Cilastatin (<1%)
Imipramine
Inamrinone (1–2%)
Indapamide (1–10%)
Infliximab (<2%)
Interferon alfa-2a (6%)
Ipratropium
Irbesartan (<1%)
Irinotecan
Isoproterenol
Isosorbide dinitrate
Isradipine (<1%)
Ivermectin
Ketamine (1–10%)
Ketoprofen (<1%)
Labetalol (1–5%)
Levodopa
Levorphanol
Lidocaine
Lisinopril (1–4%)

Lithium
Lomefloxacin (<1%)
Loratadine (<2%)
Lorazepam (1–10%)
Losartan (1–10%)
Loxapine
Maprotiline
Marihuana
Mecamylamine
Meclizine (<1%)
Mefloquine (<1%)
Melatonin
Meloxicam (<2%)
Meperidine
Mepivicaine
Meropenem (<1%)
Mesoridazine
Metaproterenol (<1%)
Metaraminol
Methocarbamol
Methoxsalen
Methylphenidate
Metoclopramide (<1%)
Metoprolol (<1%)
Mexiletine (<1%)
Midazolam (3%)
Midodrine
Milrinone (1–10%)
Mirtazapine (<1%)
Misoprostol (<1%)
Mistletoe
Mitotane
Mitoxantrone (1–10%)
Modafinil (2%)
Moexipril (1–10%)
Molindone
Moricizine (<1%)
Morphine (>10%)
Moxifloxacin (<3%)
Mycophenolate (3–20%)
Nadolol (1–10%)
Naloxone
Naproxen (<1%)
Nefazodone (1–10%)
Neostigmine
Nesiritide (11%)
Niacin
Nifedipine (5%)
Nimodipine (1–8%)
Nitroglycerin (4%)
Nortriptyline
Olanzapine (1–10%)
Ondansetron (<1%)
Oxcarbazepine (1–2%)
Oxprenolol
Oxycodone (1–10%)
Oxymorphone (>10%)
Paclitaxel
Palonosetron (1%)
Pamidronate (<1%)
Pantoprazole (<1%)
Paroxetine (<1%)
Peg-interferon alfa-2a (<1%)
Peg-interferon alfa-2b (<1%)
Pentamidine (>10%)
Pentazocine
Pentobarbital
Pentoxifylline (<1%)
Perflutren (<1%)
Pergolide (1–10%)
Perphenazine
Phendimetrazine
Phenelzine
Phenformin
Phenobarbital
Phenoxybenzamine
Phentermine
Phentolamine
Phenylephrine
Phenytoin
Physostigmine
Phytonadione
Pimozide
Pindolol (<1%)
Pramipexole (>10%)
Prazosin (1–10%)
Procainamide (<5%)
Procarbazine (<1%)

Prochlorperazine
Progesterone (<5%)
Promethazine
Propafenone
Propofol (3–26%)
Propoxyphene
Propranolol
Protamine sulfate
Protriptyline
Pyridostigmine
Quetiapine
Quinapril (3%)
Quinidine
Ramipril
Remifentanil (1–10%)
Riluzole (1–10%)
Rimantadine (1–10%)
Risperidone (1–10%)
Ritonavir (<1%)
Rituximab (1–10%)
Rivastigmine (<2%)
Rocuronium (>1%)
Ropinirole (2%)
Sargramostin (>10%)
Scopolamine
Selegiline
Sevoflurane (~1%)
Sildenafil (<2%)
Sirolimus (3–20%)
Sotalol (6%)
Sparfloxacin (<1%)
Streptokinase (>10%)
Streptomycin
Succinylcholine (1–10%)
Sufentanil (>10%)
Sulprostone
Tacrolimus (3–15%)
Tadalafil (<2%)
Tamsulosin
Tegaserod (<1%)
Tenecteplase
Terazosin (3%)
Terbutaline (1–10%)
Thalidomide
Thiopental
Thioridazine
Thiothixene
Timolol (<1%)
Tinzaparin (1–10%)
Tizanidine (>10%)
Tocainide (3%)
Tolazoline
Tolcapone (>10%)
Torsemide (<1%)
Tositumomab+Iodine I 131 (10%)
Tramadol
Tranylcypromine
Trastuzumab (<1%)
Travoprost (1–5%)
Trazodone (1–10%)
Treprostinil (4%)
Tretinoin (>10%)
Trifluoperazine
Trimethobenzamide
Trimipramine
Urokinase (<1%)
Valdecoxib (<2%)
Valsartan (7%)
Vancomycin (>10%)
Vardenafil (<2%)
Vecuronium (<1%)
Venlafaxine
Verapamil (2%)
Vinblastine (<1%)
Vincristine (1–10%)
Voriconazole (2%)
Ziprasidone (2%)
Zoledronic acid (1–10%)

MYCOCARDIAL ISCHEMIA

Adenosine
Almotriptan (<1%)
Amifostine (<1%)
Amphetamines
Anastrozole (<1%)
Beta agonists
Caffeine
Capecitabine (<5%)

Carvedilol (<1%)
Cilostazol (<2%)
Dipyridamole
Ergotamine
Etanercept (<3%)
Fluorouracil (10%)
Letrozole (<2%)
Nifedipine
Palonosetron (<1%)
Pantoprazole (<1%)
Pindolol
Rofecoxib
Sildenafil (<2%)
Sumatriptan (<1%)
Theophylline
Thyroxine
Verapamil
Vincristine
Vinblastine

MYOCARDIAL INFARCTION

Acitretin
Adalimumab (<1%)
Alemtuzumab
Almotriptan (<1%)
Amitriptyline
Aprepitant
Bortezomib
Candesartan
Captopril
Cefdinir (<1%)
Celecoxib (<2%)
Cilostazol (<2%)
Ciprofloxacin (<1%)
Clozapine (<1%)
Cyclobenzaprine (<1%)
Cyclophosphamide (1–10%)
Cyclosporine (1–10%)
Denileukin (1%)
Dihydroergotamine (<1%)
Dipyridamole (<1%)
Docetaxel (<1%)
Dofetilide (<2%)
Doxazosin (<1%)
Ephedra
Estradiol
Estramustine (1–10%)
Estrogens (conjugated)
Etanercept (<3%)
Felodipine (<1%)
Fenofibrate
Fluoxetine (<1%)
Flutamide (<1%)
Fosinopril (<1%)
Goserelin (1–10%)
Imipramine
Indinavir (<1%)
Interferon alfa-2a (1%)
Interferon alfa-2b (<5%)
Interferon beta-1b (<1%)
Irbesartan (<1%)
Isoproterenol
Letrozole (<2%)
Leuprolide
Levorphanol
Lisinopril (<1%)
Meloxicam (<1%)
Meropenem (<1%)
Mifepristone (<1%)
Milrinone (<1%)
Misoprostol (<1%)
Moexipril (<1%)
Moricizine (<1%)
Nabumetone (<1%)
Naratriptan (<1%)
Nifedipine (<1%)
Nortriptyline
Peg-interferon alfa-2a (<1%)
Pergolide (1%)
Prazosin (<1%)
Protriptyline
Quinapril (<1%)
Rabeprazole (<1%)
Ramipril (<1%)
Ritonavir (<1%)
Rizatriptan (<1%)
Tadalafil (<2%)
Tenecteplase

Tinzaparin (<1%)
Toremifene (1–10%)
Tretinoin (1–10%)
Trimipramine
Urokinase (<1%)
Valdecoxib (<2%)
Vardenafil (<)
Verapamil (<1%)
Voriconazole (<1%)

MYOCARDIAL TOXICITY

Amsacrine
Capecitabine
Cisplatin
Cyclophosphamide
Daunorubicin
Doxorubicin
Fluorouracil
Gadodiamide
Idarubicin
Influenza vaccines
Interferon alpha (5–15%)
Mitazantrone
Paclitaxel
Procainamide
Quinidine
Trastuzumab
Tricyclic antidepressants

MYOCARDITIS

Adriamycin
Anthracyclines
Co-trimoxazole
Cyclophosphamide
Daunorubicin (<1%)
Ephedra
Influenza vaccines
Mesalamine (<1%)
Methysergide
Oxybutynin
Procainamide (<1%)
Theophylline
Thiazide diuretics
Tretinoin (1–10%)

PALPITATIONS

Adenosine
Albuterol
Amiloride (<1%)
Amitriptyline
Amlodipine (1–4%)
Atropine
Baclofen (<1%)
Bisoprolol (1–10%)
Bosentan (5%)
Bupivacaine
Bupropion (5%)
Butorphanol (<1%)
Cabergoline (1%)
Candesartan
Captopril (1%)
Carteolol (1–10%)
Carvedilol (1–10%)
Cevimeline (1 10%)
Cilostazol (5–10%)
Clemastine
Clomipramine (1–10%)
Clopidogrel (1–3%)
Cromolyn
Desipramine
Desmopressin
Diltiazem (1–2%)
Diphenhydramine
Dobutamine (1–3%)
Dopamine
Doxazosin (1–2%)
Eletriptan (1–10%)
Ephedra
Ephedrine
Escitalopram (1–10%)
Famotidine (<1%)
Felbamate (1–10%)
Felodipine (2–17%)
Feverfew
Flecainide (6%)
Flumazenil (1–10%)
Fluoxetine (1–10%)
Flurazepam
Fluvoxamine (1–10%)

Fosphenytoin (<1%)
Frovatriptan (1%)
Galantamine (<1%)
Ginseng
Glatiramer (17%)
Goserelin (1–10%)
Hawthorn
Hepatitis B vaccine
Hydromorphone
Hyoscyamine
Ibutilide (1%)
Imipramine
Indapamide (1–10%)
Insulin
Interferon alfa-2a (<3%)
Interferon beta-1b (4%)
Ipratropium (2%)
Isoproterenol
Isotretinoin
Lamotrigine (<1%)
Levodopa
Levorphanol
Meclizine (<1%)
Mefloquine (<1%)
Megestrol (8%)
Meprobamate
Metaproterenol (4%)
Metaraminol
Metformin (1–10%)
Methamphetamine
Methylphenidate
Metolazone
Metoprolol
Mexiletine (4–8%)
Moexipril (<1%)
Moricizine (1–10%)
Morphine (>10%)
Mycophenolate (3–20%)
Nadolol (1–10%)
Niacin
Nicardipine (3–4%)
Nifedipine (2–7%)
Nimodipine (3%)
Nortriptyline
Oxybutynin (2–5%)
Paroxetine (1–10%)
Perflutren (<0.5%)
Pergolide (2%)
Phentermine
Physostigmine
Prazosin (5%)
Procyclidine
Protriptyline
Pseudoephedrine
Quetiapine
Quinidine (7%)
Ropinirole (3%)
Rosuvastatin (~1%)
Salmeterol (1–10%)
Scopolamine
Selegiline
Sertraline (1–10%)
Siberian ginseng
Sibutramine (1–10%)
Sotalol (14%)
Tadalafil (<2%)
Tamsulosin (<1%)
Terazosin (1–10%)
Tizanidine (1–10%)
Valproic acid (1–10%)
Valsartan (<1%)
Zolmitriptan (~2%)
Zolpidem (1–10%)

PERICARDIAL EFFUSION

Adalimumab (<5%)
Alteplase
Bortezomib
Capecitabine (<5%)
Clozapine (<1%)
Doxorubicin (1–10%)
Interferon beta-1b (<1%)
Minoxidil (<1%)
Sargramostin (4%)
Streptokinase
Tenecteplase
Trastuzumab (<1%)

PERICARDITIS

Adalimumab
Alemtuzumab
Alteplase
Aminosalicylic acid
Captopril
Cevimeline (<1%)
Clozapine (<1%)
Cytarabine (>10%)
Dantrolene (1–10%)
Daunorubicin (<1%)
Demeclocycline
Doxorubicin (1–10%)
Doxycycline
Filgrastim (<1%)
Hydralazine
Influenza vaccines
Oxytetracycline
Procainamide (<1%)
Quinupristin/Dalfopristin (<1%)
Sargramostin (<1%)
Streptokinase
Tenecteplase
Tetracycline
Tocainide (<1%)
Tretinoin (1–10%)
Valdecoxib (<2%)

QT PROLONGATION

Alfuzosin
Amantadine
Amiodarone
Amitriptyline
Aripiprazole
Artemisia
Azithromycin
Bepridil (1–10%)
Chloral hydrate
Chloroquine
Chlorpromazine
Ciprofloxacin
Cisapride
Citalopram
Clarithromycin (<1%)
Clomipramine
Disopyramide
Dobutamine
Dolasetron
Domperidone
Dopamine
Doxepin
Droperidol (>10%)
Encainide
Ephedra
Ephedrine
Epinephrine
Erythromycin
Felbamate
Flecainide
Fluconazole
Fluoxetine (<1%)
Foscarnet
Fosphenytoin (<1%)
Galantamine
Granisetron
Haloperidol
Ibutilide (1%)
Imipramine
Indapamide
Isradipine
Itraconazole
Ketoconazole
Levofloxacin
Levomepromazine
Lithium
Mefloquine
Mesoridazine
Methadone
Methylphenidate
Midodrine
Moxifloxacin (<3%)
Naratriptan
Nelfinavir (<2%)
Norepinephrine
Nortriptyline
Octreotide
Ofloxacin
Olanzapine

Ondansetron
Palonosetron
Paroxetine
Pentamidine
Phentermine
Phenylephrine
Phenylpropanolamine
Procainamide
Propranolol
Pseudoephedrine
Quetiapine
Quinidine
Rabeprazole (<1%)
Risperidone
Salbutamol
Salmeterol
Sertindole
Sertraline
Sibutramine
Sotalol
Sparfloxacin (1%)
Tacrolimus
Tamoxifen
Terbutaline
Terfenadine
Thioridazine
Tizanidine
Tocainide
Trimethoprim/Sulfamethoxazole
Trimipramine
Vardenafil
Venlafaxine
Verapamil
Voriconazole (<1%)
Ziprasidone (<1%)
Zolmitriptan (<1%)

SYNCOPE

Abarelix
Adalimumab
Alemtuzumab
Alfuzosin (<1%)
Amitriptyline
Amoxapine (<1%)
Atazanavir (<3%)
Atorvastatin (<2%)
Azithromycin (<1%)
Baclofen (<1%)
Benazepril (<1%)
Betaxolol (1–10%)
Bivalirudin (<1%)
Bretylium (<1%)
Budesonide (1–10%)
Bupropion (5%)
Butorphanol (<1%)
Cabergoline (1%)
Captopril
Carbamazepine
Carvedilol (3–8%)
Celecoxib (<2%)
Cevimeline (<1%)
Cidofovir (1–10%)
Cilostazol (<2%)
Ciprofloxacin (<1%)
Clonidine (<1%)
Clopidogrel (1–3%)
Clozapine (1–10%)
Daunorubicin (<1%)
Diltiazem (<2%)
Dinoprostone (<1%)
Dipyridamole (<1%)
Dirithromycin (1–10%)
Dofetilide (<2%)
Donepezil (1–10%)
Doxazosin (2%)
Edrophonium
Enalapril (1–2%)
Entacapone (1%)
Escitalopram (<1%)
Etodolac (<1%)
Felodipine (<1%)
Foscarnet (<1%)
Fosinopril (<1%)
Fosphenytoin (<1%)
Frovatriptan (<1%)
Galantamine (<2%)
Gemfibrozil (<1%)
Glipizide

Hepatitis B vaccine
Ibutilide (0.3%)
Infliximab (<2%)
Interferon alfa-2b (<5%)
Interferon beta-1b (<1%)
Isosorbide mononitrate (<1%)
Isotretinoin
Isradipine (<1%)
Labetalol (<1%)
Levalbuterol (<2%)
Levodopa
Lithium
Losartan (<1%)
Loxapine
Mefloquine (<1%)
Meloxicam (<1%)
Memantine (1–10%)
Meprobamate
Mesoridazine
Methadone
Methocarbamol
Metolazone
Mexiletine (<1%)
Mifepristone (1%)
Modafinil (1%)
Moexipril (<1%)
Moricizine (<1%)
Nabumetone (<1%)
Niacin
Nicardipine (<1%)
Nifedipine
Oxaliplatin
Oxcarbazepine (<1%)
Oxycodone (<1%)
Pamidronate (<6%)
Pantoprazole (<1%)
Pentazocine
Pergolide (2%)
Phenobarbital
Phenoxybenzamine
Pramipexole (1–10%)
Prazosin (1%)
Progesterone (<5%)
Propofol (<1%)
Pyridostigmine
Quinapril (<1%)
Quinidine (1–8%)
Quinupristin/Dalfopristin (<1%)
Rabeprazole (<1%)
Ramipril (<1%)
Ritonavir (<1%)
Rivastigmine (3%)
Rosuvastatin (<1%)
Sargramostin (>10%)
Selegiline
Sevoflurane (<1%)
Sibutramine
Sildenafil (<2%)
Sirolimus (3–20%)
Sodium oxybate (<1%)
Sotalol (5%)
Sumatriptan (<1%)
Tadalafil (<2%)
Tamsulosin (<1%)
Tegaserod (<1%)
Terazosin (1%)
Teriparatide (3%)
Thalidomide
Thiopental
Thiothixene
Tizanidine (1–10%)
Tocainide (<1%)
Tramadol (<1%)
Trastuzumab (<1%)
Travoprost (1–10%)
Valdecoxib (<2%)
Valsartan (<1%)
Vardenafil (<2%)
Verapamil (<1%)
Voriconazole (<1%)
Zaleplon (<1%)
Zanamivir (1.5%)
Ziprasidone (<1%)
Zolmitriptan (<1%)
Zonisamide (<1%)

TACHYCARDIA

Aconite

Alemtuzumab (11%)
Alfuzosin (<1%)
Alprostadil (1–10%)
Amiodarone
Amitriptyline
Aprepitant
Aripiprazole (1%)
Arnica
Arsenic trioxide (55%)
Atomoxetine (2%)
Atracurium (<1%)
Atropine
Basiliximab
Benztropine
Bepridil
Bethanechol
Bexarotene
Buprenorphine
Bupropion
Butorphanol
Caffeine
Captopril (1%)
Carbamazepine
Carisoprodol
Caspofungin (<2%)
Chasteberry (2–5%)
Chloroquine
Chlorpromazine
Cidofovir
Cilostazol (4%)
Cimetidine (<1%)
Cisapride (withdrawn)
Cladribine
Clemastine
Clomipramine
Clonidine
Cocaine
Codeine
Cromolyn
Cyclobenzaprine
Daclizumab
Deferoxamine
Denileukin (12%)
Desipramine
Digoxin
Dihydroergotamine
Diltiazem (<2%)
Dimercaprol (>10%)
Diphenhydramine
Dipyridamole (3%)
Dofetilide (3%)
Dopamine
Doxepin
Doxorubicin (>10%)
Dronabinol (1–10%)
Droperidol (1–10%)
Edrophonium
Eletriptan (<1%)
Ephedra
Ephedrine
Epinephrine
Ergotamine
Ertapenem
Erythromycin
Escitalopram (<1%)
Etodolac (<1%)
Etomidate (<1%)
Famotidine (<1%)
Felbamate (1–10%)
Famotidine (0.4–2%)
Fenoldopam
Fenoprofen (<1%)
Fluoxetine (<1%)
Fluphenazine
Fomepizole (1–10%)
Frovatriptan (<1%)
Gatifloxacin (<1%)
Gemtuzumab (10%)
Ginseng
Glatiramer (5%)
Glycopyrrolate (<1%)
Goserelin (1–10%)
Guarana
Haloperidol
Hepatitis B vaccine
Hydralazine
Hydromorphone
Hyoscyamine

Ibritumomab (<1%)
Ibuprofen (<1%)
Ibutilide (1%)
Imipramine
Infliximab (<2%)
Insulin
Interferon beta-1b (4%)
Ipratropium
Isoprenaline
Isoproterenol
Isosorbide dinitrate
Isosorbide mononitrate
Isotretinoin
Isradipine (1–3%)
Ivermectin
Ketamine (>10%)
Ketoprofen (<1%)
Leuprolide
Levalbuterol (<2%)
Levofloxacin (1%)
Levorphanol
Levothyroxine
Lidoflazine
Lomefloxacin (<1%)
Loratadine (<2%)
Loxapine
Mefenamic acid (<1%)
Mefloquine (<1%)
Meprobamate
Mesna (<1%)
Mesoridazine
Metaproterenol (<17%)
Metaraminol
Methamphetamine
Methylphenidate
Metoclopramide (<1%)
Minoxidil (>10%)
Mitoxantrone (<1%)
Molindone
Moxifloxacin (<3%)
Mycophenolate (20–22%)
Nadolol (<1%)
Naloxone
Neostigmine
Nesiritide (2–10%)
Niacin
Niacinamide
Nicardipine (1–3%)
Nicotine (>10%)
Nitroglycerin (<1%)
Nortriptyline
Olanzapine (1–10%)
Olmesartan (<1%)
Ondansetron (<1%)
Oxybutynin
Palonosetron (1%)
Pancuronium
Peg-interferon alfa-2b (<1%)
Pentamidine
Pentazocine
Perflutren (<0.5%)
Perphenazine
Phenothiazine
Phenoxybenzamine
Phentermine
Phentolamine
Phosphodiesterase inhibitors
Physostigmine
Pilocarpine (1–10%)
Pirbuterol (1–10%)
Pramipexole (1–10%)
Prochlorperazine
Procyclidine
Promethazine
Propofol (1–3%)
Protriptyline
Pseudoephedrine
Pyridostigmine
Quetiapine
Rabeprazole
Remifentanil (1–10%)
Riluzole (1–10%)
Risperidone (1–10%)
Rituximab
Rivastigmine (<2%)
Ropinirole (2%)
Salmeterol (1–10%)
Sargramostin (>10%)

Scopolamine
Selegiline
Sevoflurane (~1%)
Siberian ginseng
Sotalol
St John's wort
Succinylcholine (1–10%)
Tadalafil (<2%)
Terazosin (1–10%)
Terbutaline (1–10%)
Thiothixene
Tinzaparin (1–10%)
Tocainide (3%)
Tolterodine (<1%)
Trastuzumab (5%)
Trazodone (<1%)
Trihexyphenidyl
Trimipramine
Urokinase (<1%)
Valdecoxib (<2%)
Valproic acid (1–10%)
Vardenafil (<2%)
Vecuronium (<1%)
Venlafaxine (2%)
Verapamil (1%)
Vinblastine (<1%)
Vincamine
Vincristine (1–10%)
Voriconazole (3%)
Yohimbine
Ziprasidone (2%)

THROMBOPHLEBITIS

Alemtuzumab (<1%)
Carbamazepine
Cefamandole (1–10%)
Cefoxitin (<1%)
Celecoxib (<2%)
Cevimeline (<2%)
Eletriptan (<1%)
Esmolol (<1%)
Etanercept (<3%)
Filgrastim (<1%)
Flutamide (<1%)
Fosphenytoin (<1%)
Furosemide
Infliximab (<2%)
Irinotecan (1–10%)
Letrozole (<2%)
Mephobarbital (<1%)
Octreotide (<1%)
Pantoprazole (<1%)
Pentostatin (<1%)
Rivastigmine (<2%)
Saquinavir (<1%)
Sargramostin (<1%)
Tacrolimus (3–15%)

TORSADES DE POINTES

Adenosine
Alfuzosin
Amantadine
Amiodarone
Amitriptyline
Antiarrhythmics class 1A
Antiarrhythmics class III
Arsenic
Astemizole (withdrawn)
Azithromycin (<1%)
Bepridil
Celecoxib
Chloral hydrate
Chloroquine
Chlorpromazine
Cisapride (withdrawn)
Citalopram
Clarithromycin
Clindamycin
Co-trimoxazole
Desipramine
Disopyramide
Dofetilide (3%)
Dolasetron
Domperidone
Droperidol (<1%)
Erythromycin
Escitalopram (<1%)
Felbamate

Fluconazole
Fluoxetine (<1%)
Fluvoxamine (<1%)
Foscarnet
Fosphenytoin
Ganciclovir (<1%)
Gatifloxacin (<1%)
Gemifloxacin
Granisetron
Halofantrine
Haloperidol
Ibutilide (2%)
Imipramine
Indapamide
Isradipine
Itraconazole
Ketoconazole
Levofloxacin (<1%)
Lithium
Loratadine
Maprotiline
Mefloquine
Mesoridazine
Methadone
Mexiletine (<1%)
Milrinone
Mirtazapine (<1%)
Moexipril
Moxifloxacin (<3%)
Nelfinavir (<2%)
Nicardipine
Octreotide
Ofloxacin
Olanzapine
Ondansetron
Paroxetine (<1%)
Pentamidine
Pimozide
Procainamide
Quetiapine
Quinidine
Quinine
Risperidone
Salmeterol
Sertraline
Sibutramine (<1%)
Sotalol
Sparfloxacin
Tacrolimus
Tamoxifen
Telithromycin
Terfenadine (withdrawn)
Terodiline
Thioridazine
Tizanidine
Vardenafil
Venlafaxine
Voriconazole (<1%)
Ziprasidone

VENTRICULAR FIBRILLATION

Acebutolol (<1%)
Alemtuzumab (<1%)
Almotriptan (<1%)
Bivalirudin (<1%)
Digoxin
Dihydroergotamine (<1%)
Dofetilide (<0.4%)
Dopamine
Erythromycin
Filgrastim (<1%)
Flecainide (<1%)
Isradipine (<1%)
Labetalol (<1%)
Milrinone (1–10%)
Naratriptan (<1%)
Paroxetine (<1%)
Procainamide (<1%)
Quinidine (<1%)
Scopolamine

VENTRICULAR TACHYCARDIA

Abciximab
Alemtuzumab (<1%)
Almotriptan (<1%)
Alprostadil (1–10%)
Alteplase
Amiodarone (1–10%)

Argatroban (5%)
Azithromycin (<1%)
Clarithromycin (<1%)
Dihydroergotamine (<1%)
Dipyridamole (<1%)
Dofetilide (3%)
Droperidol (<1%)
Fluoxetine (<1%)
Fluvoxamine (<1%)
Galantamine (<1%)
Glycopyrrolate (<1%)
Ibutilide (2%)
Levofloxacin (<1%)
Moricizine (<1%)
Moxifloxacin (<3%)
Naratriptan (<1%)
Nesiritide (3%)
Nizatidine (<1%)
Paroxetine (<1%)
Quinidine (<1%)
Ropinirole
Sertraline (<1%)
Streptokinase
Torsemide (<1%)
Voriconazole (<1%)
Zaleplon (<1%)